Anass Sentissi

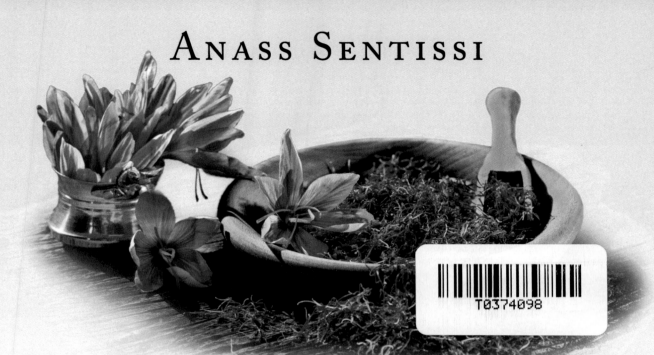

SAFFRON
FOR ALL
SEASONS

Holistic Recipes for Optimum
Health & Jubilant Wellness

Order this book online at www.trafford.com
or email orders@trafford.com

Most Trafford titles are also available at major online book retailers.

Print information available on the last page.

ISBN: 978-1-4907-9236-1 (sc)
          978-1-4907-9235-4 (e)

Library of Congress Control Number: 2018965402

Our mission is to efficiently provide the world's finest, most comprehensive book publishing service, enabling every author to experience success. To find out how to publish your book, your way, and have it available worldwide, visit us online at www.trafford.com

Trafford rev. 04/29/2019

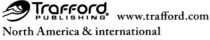

www.trafford.com
North America & international
toll-free: 1 888 232 4444 (USA & Canada)
fax: 812 355 4082

Saffron for All Seasons

"My profession is to be forever journeying—to travel about the Universe so that I may know all its conditions."

~Avicenna 10th-11th Century

Table of Contents

The Moroccan Cuisine an Enrichment of the Healthy Mediterranean Diet

I've had many professions and worn many hats throughout the course of my life, but perhaps my most prized profession, my highest calling—also the professed by Persian scholar and prolific polymath Avicenna—is the perpetual journey towards a greater understanding of the Universe. Along this journey, I've come to see that everything in the Universe is connected. From music and math to medicine and metaphysics, from poetry and psychology to astronomy and art, from the individual and the environment to the Earth and the Universe that surrounds it, all of existence is interwoven in the tapestry of life.

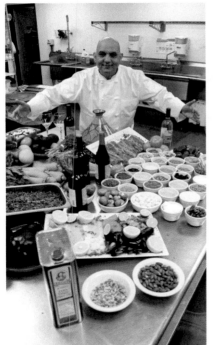

Executive Chef and Owner of two Indianapolis restaurants (downtown Indy favorites— Saffron Cafe, serving authentic & traditional made-from-scratch Moroccan-Mediterranean cuisine and Poccadio Moroccan Grill & Gourmet Sandwiches, serving healthy Moroccan favorites on the go). Chef Sentissi is a self-made entrepreneur on a quest to popularize healthy eating 'on the go' in today's market—Moroccan style!

Chef Sentissi is often described as a modern-day Renaissance Man. He is not only a fresh food enthusiast with a passion for nurturing you with his very tasty and artful array of herbs and spices, he is also known for concocting memorable and nourishing inventions like his famous Spicy Orange & Avocado. The Chef is also a lover of art, science, metaphysics, health and healing.

Chef Sentissi is an accomplished percussionist and performer of Andalusian music. He teaches Sunday Cooking Classes where he shares his love of Moroccan cooking, culture and history, along with power point presentation on nutrition science.

Chef Sentissi focuses on herbs and spices and use of Saffron to achieve a depth of flavor in his recipes that when consumed, create balance in the body. Sentissi is an artist and his medium is food. He prepares his fresh, all-natural ingredients by putting into practice his study of each spice and each herb and their various combinations to produce wholesome and fulfilling dishes which yield that perfect 'picture' of health.

Often quoting Hippocrates, "Let thy food be thy medicine, and thy medicine be thy food", Chef Sentissi believes 'you are what you eat'. Sentissi's recipes are packed full of vitamins, nutrients, and anti-oxidants as well as super anti-inflammatory saffron and garlic. Sentissi's menus boast a plethora of vegetarian, vegan, and gluten-free options as well as all hormone-free and halal (or Kosher) meats. The best part of eating healthy at Saffron Cafe or Poccadio is that everything tastes amazing.

Chef Sentissi somehow finds a way to incorporate all his knowledge, understanding, and love for each of his passions into everything he does and graciously shares himself and his magnificent food with everyone he encounters. That is why eating something prepared by (or with) Chef Sentissi is an epicurean adventure sure to delight your senses. It is a given that "when you try it...you will love it!"

The mission of this book is to educate the world to nurture both body and mind by practicing the philosophy of eating wholesome foods. By eating mindfully, people can look forward to profound health, jubilant wellness, and sheer vitality.

A highly successful nutritional philosophy is yours for the taking. As soon as you know why eating whole foods is important and what various ingredients can be used for, you will have a better appreciation for the foods you eat and be able to make better decisions regarding what goes onto your plate.

I'm the chef at the Saffron Café in Indianapolis, Indiana. Saffron, as you may have guessed, is my favorite ingredient because of the flavor as well as the health benefits. Saffron can be used throughout all seasons to create amazing meals that are good for the mind, body and soul. With the use of other ingredients, it's a great way to ensure that you are eating well – and making sure that your family is getting the nutrition they need to grow healthy and strong.

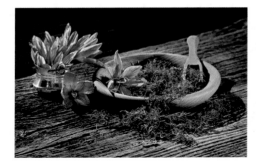

Chapter 1: Why Eating Whole Foods Can Change Your Life's Energy

You are probably reading this eBook because you want to begin eating healthier. You may have an array of goals – losing weight, feeling healthier, looking better, or any number of other goals.

The main question that you probably have is: *How will eating whole foods change your life's energy?* There are various ways to answer this question. First, you have to know that your body is different from everyone else's body and what you fuel your body with affects the amount of energy that you have.

How do I get more energy?

How do I lose weight?

How do I pay attention to the needs of my body?

How do I support the local economy?

How Do I Improve My Overall Level Of Health?

All of these questions can be answered in the same way. **Eat more whole foods!** By doing so, you will slowly start to change the energy in your life because you are feeding your body the vitamins and nutrients that it needs to not only survive but also to thrive.

Let's take a look at what processed foods are doing to your body. Any time you buy food that is already prepared into something else, it is processed. It can be canned, bagged, frozen, shrink-wrapped, or served up at a restaurant. It's not a "whole food" and it's not good for your body.

There are plenty of reasons why you should say goodbye to processed foods.

1. They're more expensive
2. Pesticides are found in the food
3. It will reduce your lifespan
4. It can result in accelerated aging
5. The chemicals can have negative impacts on your organs
6. The additives only make you hungrier
7. Low-fat foods are stripped of the healthy fats that help you
8. Food coloring makes food look fresher than it really is
9. Added sugar can be as addictive as drugs
10. Processed foods can result in inflammation

Over 80,000 different chemicals have been approved to be used in the United States. When you eat any kind of processed food, you could be consuming a large number of these chemicals. The scary part is that only 15 percent or so have been tested for a long-term impact on humans. This means that your guess as to the long-term effect of these chemicals are as good a guess as anyone else's.

If you have ever bought processed meats or flavored noodle mixes, there are high levels of phosphate-focused ingredients inside. These can be responsible for deteriorating your kidneys and weakening your bones. If you see sodium phosphate on the label of a food that you really want, think again. You want to avoid anything with *"phos"* in the name.

When you look at health problems just with a single ingredient of processed food, it's easy to see why you should be sticking with whole foods instead of exploring the "easy" way and buying the processed foods.

Low-fat products are bought in bulk by people who want to lose weight. Research has shown that this fad **has only lead to higher levels of obesity**. The reason is because in the processing of the food, the healthy fat known as conjugated linoleic acid is stripped away. This fat is what is responsible for fighting cancer as well as weight gain. You need this fat and instead, the processed foods are replacing it with more sugar, and that's not helping you in any way.

Virtually all that can go wrong with the body is a result of inflammation. Research has shown that processed foods have a higher ability to create inflammation in the body. This is why children will develop asthma after eating large amounts of fast food and why some people develop digestive problems by eating too much processed meats and meals.

If processed foods are not the answer, what is? Whole foods are the way to go. They are plant-based and generally healthier for you because they haven't been tampered with by tens of thousands of chemicals. It is simply the food that you are eating, making it easier for your body to digest.

Eating whole foods will make you feel healthier. If you are constantly eating foods that contain chemicals, it can affect the way your skin feels, how your body digests, and how much energy you are actually getting. Plant-based products have higher levels of vitamins and minerals, which will replenish your body and give you more energy, better looking skin, and a faster digestive tract. All of this is going to impact how you feel on a day to day basis.

Research has shown that various chronic conditions have been assisted or even reversed by adopting a diet that consists of whole foods. This includes diseases such as diabetes, high blood pressure, IBS, heart disease, and cancer.

You can also become a better athlete when you aren't putting so many chemicals in your body. The food dyes and the phosphates in processed foods along with everything else can make you feel sluggish. Your joints may be inflamed and you may not be able to get the level of oxygen into your lungs as you need. Endurance can be improved when you get rid of the processed foods.

It's also possible to have a better impact on the earth. It takes more energy (and everything else) to produce animal products than it does to produce plants. This means that farming will be more sustainable with an emphasis on plant-based products.

You also have the keen ability to control everything that goes into your body. If you eat processed foods, you never know exactly **what** you are eating. Look at the box of food that you are about to prepare for your family. Can you even pronounce all of the ingredients? Do you know what half of them are? Have you heard of all of them before? Do you think they grown naturally in the earth? If you have doubts about the ingredients, then why eat them? You can rule out the uncertainty of the foods that you eat by focusing on whole foods. If you make a stew using water, spices, and fresh vegetables, those are the ingredients, plain and simple.

Whether you look at the reasons not to eat processed foods or you look at the reasons why you should eat whole foods, the outcome is the same. There is the undeniable conclusion that whole foods are simply the better thing to put inside your body.

Chapter 2: Why Diets Don't Work for Everyone

If you have ever gone on a diet that someone else was on, you know that the results can vary dramatically. Some people cut out carbs and have amazing results. Other people cut out fat or protein and have amazing results. Not everyone is able to get amazing results with every diet that's out there and it all has to do with your DNA makeup.

What you eat is metabolized in your body in a unique way. Some people have higher metabolisms than others. You may have noticed this by the amount of food that a person eats with little to no impact on the amount of weight that they gain. You may be one of those fortunate individuals or you may not. Either way, this is going to impact how certain diets affect you.

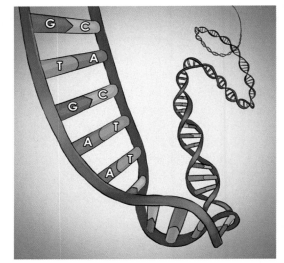

There are some ways to speed up your metabolism so that you burn more calories. Eating balanced meals throughout the day, having protein for breakfast, lunch and dinner, and choosing organic produce are all ways to help you.

With this in mind, there are certain aspects to diets that will work for anyone. Working out and making healthy food decisions are the ultimate way to lose weight, regardless of how much you have to lose or what trend may be out there for dieting.

The term "diet" has gotten a bad reputation. You may not actually need to go on a diet in the typical sense of the word. Instead, you need to pay attention to what you eat and change your overall way of looking at food. As you understand bio-identifiable theory and the top ingredients that you should cook with, you will see how eating healthier is going to impact your overall well-being.

Diets don't work for everyone because each person needs different levels of nutrition. You may be pre-disposed to allergic reactions and sensitivities when you eat certain foods. Your digestive tract may lack certain bacteria that allow you to process the food. You may be in a region where it is easier or harder to come by certain foods.

Diets also don't work because there is a behavioral relapse that causes you to go off the diet. You are surrounded by cultural and commercial pressures to eat all sorts of different foods. These foods should be avoided once you identify what is in them and what makes them so bad for you. However, identifying these substances makes it easier for you to make more permanent modifications to your eating behaviors.

The way you store fat and how you produce and use insulin is going to affect how a diet works for you as well. Some people produce more insulin than they need while others don't produce enough. If your body isn't using the insulin as it should, it can result in the cells storing fat instead of using it for energy, which is going to result in weight gain.

The more you understand your body, the easier it will be to determine the diet that will actually work for you. This comes back to the holistic approach when creating a lifestyle change with the foods that you eat. It's hard to look at one aspect of your body without looking at the whole thing because everything is interconnected.

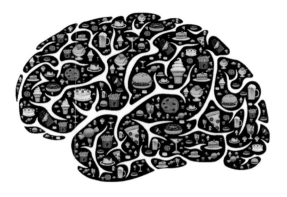

You also have to look at what is really feeding you. As a graduate from the Institute for Integrative Nutrition, I agree completely with Joshua Rosenthal's theory on bio-individuality and primary food. Primary food is what feeds you, but it's not going to come on a plate.

What is primary food, then? It is the open relationships, the spiritual practice, the physical activity, and the inspiring career that feeds your soul as well as your hunger for living. These all constitute as primary foods and the more of these you get, the less you depend on secondary foods. These two are linked tightly. When you depend more on secondary foods, the primary foods that you indulge upon are reduced. If you have ever eaten as a way of making yourself feel better, you are filling yourself with secondary foods instead of turning to primary foods as you should.

By gaining a greater awareness for primary foods, you can reduce the amount of secondary foods, thus ensuring that you are a healthier, happier person. If you have ever been in love, you were all about being in the moment. You were high on life and you forgot about food. Secondary food is simply a secondary form of energy.

If you put primary food first, you can make sure that a diet (or a change in food lifestyle) is effective regardless of what your DNA is. It's also the best way to make sure that your entire life is going in a positive direction. Why focus solely on the food that you chew when you can focus on all of the food that is going to impact your life? That's the whole reason that taking a holistic approach is important. When you begin eating the right foods in every way, you will see a dramatic improvement within your life.

Chapter 3: What is the Bio-Identifiable Theory

There are many ancient philosophies that are still prevalent today. For example, Avicenna was a Persian philosopher that wrote a total of five books, completed in the year 1025. His works have helped to influence various other philosophies including Ayurvedic and Chinese medicine.

Avicenna believed in the four elements (Earth, Water, Air, and Fire) and felt that a blend of the four were important to one's health. The food that people ate was a reflection of these elements and eating too much of one and not enough of another could be damaging to one's health. Food was more than something that nourishes – and that still holds true today.

Chinese medicine, Ayurveda, and what is commonly referred to as "alternative" medicine all take the same basic approach when it comes to healing. The entire body is healed rather than focusing on a single symptom. Looking at what a person is eating is often a clue as to why they are not doing so well. If a person lacks energy, it could be as a result of digestion problems – and this is again something that comes back to the food being eaten.

Not everyone can eat the same foods because not everyone has the same level of digestion. Some people have food sensitivities and allergies. While there has been research to show that the body can be trained to overcome allergies and sensitivities, many people simply prefer to stay away from these foods – and this is fine.

When food is being avoided, it can lead to deficiencies. This is why it is of the utmost importance to learn what foods have what health benefits. For example, if a person is allergic to milk, they are not going to get the necessary levels of Vitamin D. This does not mean they simply live without Vitamin D – they simply need to locate another type of food that contains a high level of the vitamin as an acceptable substitute.

It all comes down to how everyone is different. There is such thing as Bio-Identifiable Theory. This essentially means that everyone is different in their makeup. While DNA is the same in many areas, it varies in other areas. It's what makes us unique as human beings. It's also the reason why there are so many different types of foods out there – not everyone eats all of it.

You have a unique DNA sequence, a unique set of fingerprints, and you are unique in the way that you digest food because of the various strands of bacteria that you have or don't have inside of your digestive tract.

As science becomes more advanced, it's easier to determine what a person's chemical makeup is and what sets them apart from everyone else. Scientists have been able to identify specific areas of DNA to tell them about a person's health, physical appearance and much more. While there have been many breakthroughs in modern science, we still have a long way to go in order to get a read out on exactly what is hiding within our genes.

Biological identification is a hot topic within the world of science for many reasons. People want to learn about the roles of DNA to see how things can be changed and improved upon. Those with diseases want to learn what it is about their DNA that makes them sick.

Reverse engineering is now being done based upon what is known of the human body and how it works. This allows biological relationships to be understood in greater detail and get a better understanding of metabolic networks. This allows nutritionists and doctors alike to make recommendations in terms of what a person should eat based upon such things as:

- Genetic mutations
- Blood pressure and other test results
- Current weight and desired weight
- Blood sugar levels

All of these characteristics can vary from person to person and this is the science behind why everyone needs to eat different foods. To put it another way, look at how you eat versus the way that your kids eat. They are going to eat all sorts of fattening and fried foods. Their metabolism works so fast that they will never see it as weight gain. If you were to eat like that, you would see the effects within a few weeks, most likely. As you age, your metabolism slows down and you must be more conscientious of the foods that you eat.

As you learn more about your bio-identity, you can also make better choices as to the foods that you eat. If you learn that you have high blood sugar levels, you know that you need to reduce the amount of sugary foods that you eat. If you learn that you have a sensitivity to dairy, you want to avoid eating mass amounts of milk and cheese.

Bio-individuality, your lifestyle, your general preferences, and even your ancestral background allows you to focus on the foods that you know and love. Being honest about your roots as well as how you operate from day to day is critical when establishing foods that are going to work for you. Some people have the opportunity to cook a fresh meal for dinner while others don't.

There is no universal right answer – there is only the right answer that is best for you!

It becomes more about learning how to balance the foods that you love versus the foods that you *should* have. Knowing the ingredients that you should choose from can help you immensely.

Remember that in addition to the foods that you should and shouldn't be eating based upon what your body needs, you also have cravings that may or may not push you in the right general direction.

Health coaching can make all the difference in the world. You learn how to set and accomplish goals and achieve a happy balance between your ideal weight and the foods you want to eat so that you can experience a nutritional lifestyle change that you can actually live with. As you learn about new foods, you can add new flavors to your dinner table and have more fun with the foods that you cook with.

Once you begin eating the foods that are right for you, you will find that you have more energy, more enthusiasm in the kitchen, and generally feel better about yourself!

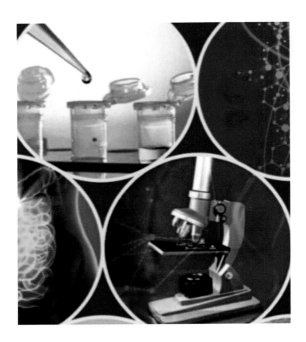

Chapter 4: Top Ingredients That Should Be in the Foods You Eat and Why

There are lists and lists of ingredients that should be in the foods that you use. How do you know which foods you should be eating? Your body is always going to seek balance. When it is out of balance, you have to listen to the subtle cues that your body gives you so that you know what ingredients should be in the foods that you are consuming.

If you are craving salt, it is your body's way of telling you that you need more zinc.

If you are constipated, it is your body's way of telling you that you need more fiber.

All sorts of signs are being given to you, so you don't need a doctor to tell you what you need to eat. You simply need to listen to your body. When you know what whole foods you should be feeding it, you can discover an array of meals to create so that you can replenish your body, provide it with energy, and encourage it to reach a healthy balance once again.

Phytonutrient Rich Foods

A plant-rich diet is going to provide you with an array of phytonutrients. These are critical to your diet because they can help to prevent a number of medical conditions ranging from high blood pressure to cancer. FDA approval has to be obtained on any claims of health benefits, though there are plenty of the benefits to go around.

Various foods contain various phytochemicals. Each phytochemical has an array of medical properties and some of them are listed below.

Curcumin: Reduces swelling, responsible for reducing effects of arthritis. Found in Turmeric.

Glucosinolates: Can stimulate antioxidant systems of the body. Found in broccoli, horseradish, and cabbage.

Anthocyanidins: Reduces the risk of coronary heart disease and can decrease lipid accumulation. Found in berries and black rice

Saponins: Can lower the blood cholesterol levels. Found in beans, quinoa, and yucca

Quercetin: Works as an anti-inflammatory and antihistamine. Found in onions, apples, grapefruit, and black tea.

There are various other foods that are high in helpful phytochemicals including:

- Gingerole (ginger)
- Kaempferol (strawberries, broccoli)
- Rutin (parsley, lemons)
- Allicin (garlic)
- Phytosterols (nuts, seeds)
- Betasitosterols (avocados, rice brown)
- Silymarin (artichokes, milk thistle)

When you cook with these ingredients, you gain the health benefits from them all.

Sea Vegetables

Did you know that sea vegetables can have 10 times or more minerals than those found on land? They are high in the minerals that your body needs, such as iron, calcium, and iodine. There are plenty of health claims to say that eating sea vegetables can help detoxify and alkalize the body as well as the remove radiation residue and lower your cholesterol.

Examples of sea vegetables include algae (spirulina), wakame, kelp, nori, and Chlorella (another type of algae).

Prebiotics

There are some foods known as prebiotics, which aren't digested by the human body. They help with digestion, but for the other foods that are consumed as a help for all of the microbes that are in your gut. It's a good idea to include certain foods in this category on a regular basis so that you can promote a higher level of health. Foods in this category include:

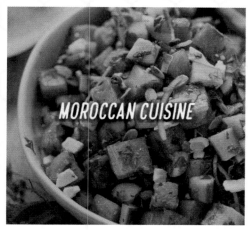

Asparagus

Chicory

Dandelion root

Leeks

Onions

Rutabaga

Some people refer to these vegetables as the building blocks because of their support of gastrointestinal health.

Probiotics

There are all sorts of foods that are good for you. In addition to raw ingredients such as fruits and vegetables, there are some others that you want to consider eating as well. Yogurt and fermented vegetables should be incorporated into your diet on occasion because they are a good source for probiotics.

What are probiotics?

They are bacteria that can help to maintain the natural balance of microflora in your intestines. There are around 400 types of probiotic bacteria in your digestive tract and they are responsible for promoting healthy digestion. Some are responsible for dealing with lactic acid while others are responsible for dealing with other things introduced into your system. Many food allergies and sensitivities stem from not having the necessary level of probiotics. Therefore, when you eat foods that contain the bacteria, you give your body's immune the boost that it needs to keep your digestive tract functioning at a high level.

Probiotics are necessary because there are all sorts of inadequate food sources that enter our bodies that lead to poor digestion. They not only confuse the digestive tract but also confuse us metabolically and within enzymatic processes. Such foods include unrated animal fats, hydrogenated oils, processed and preserved foods, gluten, sugar, and artificial sweeteners. Our bodies were created to break down what is natural. When something is unnatural, it leads to a variety of health problems.

Alkaline Foods

For a quick lesson on pH, it matters when you are talking about the foods that you eat. Low pH levels are classified as acidic and result in a greater risk of diseases such as heart disease and type 2 diabetes as well as obesity. On the other side, alkaline or high pH levels are linked to improvements in cognition and memory, so it's easy to see that you want to be eating foods that are more alkaline than acidic.

The pH scale goes from 0 to 14 with 7 being the magic number to differentiate acidic from alkaline. Some of the higher alkaline foods that you should integrate into your diet include: cucumbers, dandelion greens, eggplant, endive, mushrooms, garlic, pumpkin, tomatoes, and wild greens.

Seafood and Fish

There is a reason why you see salmon on so many different diets. It's high in Omega 3 fatty acids, along with various other types of seafood and fish. The reason that Omega 3 is such a big deal is because it reduces inflammation within the body. This can result in a variety of health benefits, including lowered blood pressure and a reduction of asthma symptoms.

Create a Nutritious Plate

I have taken a unique approach to the foods that are on my menu at the Saffron Café as well as to those that I coach. It's all about creating a nutritious plate that utilizes organic and local produce, high quality proteins, whole grains, fats that are plant-based, and water.

Learning about what a plate should look like at meal time is important so you know whether you have hit the mark or not. There should always be an emphasis on portions as well as *proportions*. As soon as you know what a nutritious plate looks like, you can repeat it again and again. If you sit down at my restaurant, you will see what one looks like. You can also learn how to make them on your own by having a key understanding of the ingredients that go into the foods that you are cooking with.

What happens when you consume a nutritious plate?

You feel better! Food isn't just about nourishment. It's a whole-body approach to help balance your body and ensure that your organs are all performing at the level that they should be. When your body is balanced you are balanced. It will influence various factors within your life including your relationships, your career, and the amount of physical activity that you do on a daily basis.

Healthy foods results in a healthy body and a healthy life!

CHAPTER 5: The Glycemic Index

The glycemic index, commonly abbreviated as GI, is a form of measurement for carbohydrate-containing foods. It ultimately measures the impact of the carbohydrates on blood sugar. This is a relatively new way of analyzing foods and is especially important for people who are diabetic – or prone to low/high blood sugar.

Prior to the glycemic index, meal plans were designed to improve blood sugar by way of analyzing the total number of carbohydrates within the foods. GI takes us to a new level by looking at how the foods will impact the blood sugar. This allows foods to be ranked as very low, low, medium, or high within the glycemic index. Many foods inside of recipe books as well as in restaurants are now identified by their glycemic index value.

GI is measured by looking at the amount of food that will provide 50 grams of available carbohydrates.

Depending upon the type of food, the portion size will vary dramatically. Available carbohydrates are defined as those that get digested and metabolized by the body easily. These are the ones that have the greatest impact on blood sugar levels. Another type of carbohydrate is that of insoluble fibers, which has virtually no immediate impact on blood sugar levels because they are not being digested readily.

After 50 grams of available carbohydrates are inside the body, blood sugar levels are then measured over a two-hour time period. In addition to this calculation, the results are placed onto a graph to summarize what is known as glucose AUC or area under the curve. The information is then taken a step further and compared to the results of either white bread or glucose. All of the numbers are given a value in comparison to white bread or glucose (which is given the value of 100 for purposes of comparison). As such, every food will have a glycemic index number ranging from 0 to 100. Those that are higher are going to have a greater impact on blood sugar levels.

Why is Glycemic Index so important?

Many people have heard about the glycemic index, but don't actually know why they should care about it. Low Glycemic Index diets have been able to impact a person's health in a number of positive ways. Those who choose lower   Glycemic Index foods have been able to reduce their risk for type II diabetes, stroke, depression, the formation of gallstones, chronic kidney disease, cardiovascular disease, the formation of uterine fibroids, breast, colon, prostate, and pancreas cancer, and much more.

Whole and natural foods are generally lower on the glycemic index, then processed foods – just another reason why you should remove processed foods from the grocery list that you use on a weekly basis.

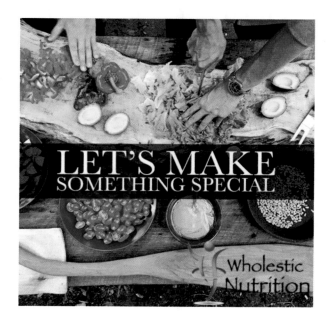

Chapter 6: The Power of Saffron

Saffron is a powerful spice that is made from the dried stigmas of the saffron plant. It takes tens of thousands of blossoms to create a single pound of the spice and that is why it is one of the most expensive spices on the planet. The good news is that it is packed with a lot of flavor, so a little bit goes a long way. Traditionally, the "threads" of saffron are added into recipes one at a time.

Many people use saffron for cooking because of all of the health benefits associated with it. There is no single use – and people from all parts of the world have been benefiting from the spice for thousands of years. It can help with:

- Infertility
- Premature ejaculation
- PMS
- Heartburn
- Dry skin
- Depression
- Intestinal gas
- Asthma
- Sleep problems
- Cancer
- Shock
- Much more!

As you can clearly see, using saffron is a great product to have within your arsenal of spices. It can also be incorporated with an array of other ingredients to create incredible dishes as well as to gain the maximum level of health benefits.

When you go to the store to buy saffron, it can be found under various names. This includes: Autumn Crocus, Indian Saffron, Spanish Saffron, Kashmira, and Kesar. Regardless of the name, it has the same effects and can be used. Be prepared to spend a lot for it, but remember that it is used in very small amounts to have a **big impact** on the dish that you are preparing.

Saffron can be used in risotto, paella, and bouillabaisse to name a few. Due to the rich yellow color, it is commonly used to color rice. You will only want to use a small amount and much of this has to do with the somewhat musty flavor of honey that can be found when you use too much.

You will find that saffron can be paired with an array of other ingredients and that's why it can be used throughout all seasons. It pairs well with seafood, rice, eggplant, beef, cinnamon, coffee, molasses, and various types of sweets. You can use the ingredient to prepare sweet and savory dishes, allowing you to create virtually anything to present on the dinner table.

We are all bombarded today with information about healthy eating but there is no decline in the rates of food-related, chronic diseases as one would expect.

The information and advice we are confronted with is inconsistent and contradictory. One day we are told to avoid fats or proteins, the next day not to eat carbohydrates. The result is that we do not trust advices about our nutrition anymore and specifically when the latest discovery in food research is not only about the food but that food can also act as a medicine.

We are not too wrong for maintaining a healthy skepticism. If we keep some basic rules in our daily diets like eating a variety of foods like whole grains, vegetables and fruits while avoiding too much candy and chocolates; and instead of drinking too many sugar saturated sodas, drink lots of plain water in between. If we do regularly participate in some physical activity—walking a few miles to the next convenience store and instead of taking the elevator in the office climb a few flights up the stairs we will feel better for having done so.

So why do we want to focus your attention to all this nutritional advice anyhow? Why if we are getting puzzled about the mostly contradictory food studies and fall in with the next trendy diet where we already know it will end in the usual Yoyo effect? Deep inside we know we will make only somebody richer following this newest trend but we are too insecure about what kind and amount of food is right for us. It is far easier to read about what we should do than really change our nutrition patterns. The bathroom scale tells us brutally and incorruptible the sins of our eating and drinking binge the day before. So, what is the problem with our regular diets?

Are we not a highly developed society where everything is only researched for our best? Sometimes we wonder how people in the "third world" areas are able to survive without supermarkets filled with conveniently packaged foods so carefully processed that nothing than only the real nutrients like pure carbohydrates are left over. All the "waste" like fibers and skins are removed in a way that our digestive system has nothing to do any more.

No taste? A few grams of taste enhancers in form of cheap glutamates or artificially propagated yeasts fake our taste buds to believe we are getting wholesome food. So far has the development of modern food gone that more than two thirds of our calories are coming just from four varieties of nutrients: Rice, wheat, soybean and corn.

This is not the food our poor brethren in developing countries are eating—their rice is rough and not polished like ours. Wheat is the only grain left over from other much rougher cereals like rye and barley, soybeans become more and more the main source of protein. And the research of the corn industry has made this crop a universal source of sugars, it replaces barley malts in beer and what they sell as maple syrup for our pancakes is often a high fructose sugar made from corn and the maple flavor is sotolon, a chemical from the family of the lactones.

We are told that to reduce the former wide variety of crops to only a few basic essential food groups is a necessity to feed the masses and as we see with corn and soy the research of the big food companies like Monsanto and Nestle can mimic the most of the older foods our parents loved so much and therefore we drink beer and maple syrup made from corn and eat tofu burgers made from soybeans.

There is nothing wrong with the food above if we integrate a tofu burger once in a while in your diet. Corn beer usually with a lower alcohol content will not kill us it just tastes terrible. The problem is that future generations will forget the taste of the real foods with original flavors and healthy roughness that our ancestors prepared.

And when it comes to foods in the developing countries we must not feel sorry for the people there, as long they have enough to eat every day, they eat the healthier foods and the civilization diseases like obesity and consequent heart attacks are occurring at a lower rate in these countries. So enough of a statement for now about the food trends in our highly sophisticated world.

If we really want to live a better and healthier life we are able to do so. Obviously the hectic existence we are living feigns us into believing that eating is only a matter of getting the energy to survive. There are no cars that repeatedly get filled up with the same gasoline over and over again.

Even animals prefer a change of their diets once in a while and you can see how happy horses are when they are able to eat sometimes fresh grasses with lots of aromatic herbs instead of the usual old dusty hay from the last summer's harvest.

Food is not only a matter of energy, but it will also provide the fine tuning to the organism we call our body as long we are prepared to listen and take efforts to learn what is best for us.

Eating in previous times was a celebration which took care for the needs of bodies, minds and spirits.

Inviting a spouse, the whole family, private or business friends to a restaurant known for its special, fresh and good food is always remembered as a treat. It is no wonder that the most business connections and business deals are done in the course of a good meal. A good dish with a bottle of wine just brings people closer they will have something to talk about aside from the business and become mutual friends. The connection between the food we eat and the influence it has on our health.

Without a doubt, as written before, our body needs food to function well. Aside from the energy it provides, the kind of food we eat gives the body signals which triggers all the metabolic processes. If metabolic processes get out of control our health declines. A good example is the consumption of alcohol. It is proven in many studies that in the Mediterranean area the usual daily one glass of red wine with a meal can prevent strokes.

However, a bottle of red wine a day with about 120 grams (4 ounces) of pure alcohol will destroy the liver with a cirrhosis in a short period of time. The *good* information given to the liver with one glass is turned to the *worst* one by stressing the functions of our body's chemical factory.

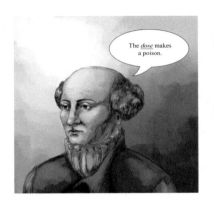

The *dose* makes a poison.

The Swiss scientist and physiologist Philip von Hohenheim (1493-1541), better known better as Paracelsus is mostly famous for his quote: Dosis Facit Venenum (The Dose Makes a Poison).

It can be perfectly translated into the upper example: while the 25 grams of alcohol once in a while is good and rejuvenating for our body, the quadruple amount of a bottle every day is poison which kills not only the liver.

Fats are the carriers of the taste as in the fatty acids the aromas are dissolved and resorbed best. In low doses fats provide for cell protection. It should be allowed to speculate here that nature is forcing us to eat fat by providing tasty aromas to eat it to give our cells enough protection. Large doses of fat are causing scaling of the arteries, they stop the metabolism of carbohydrates into direct energy and cause of heart attacks and strokes which can kill us instantly.

Our ancestors had the opposite problem they were seldom able to provide sufficient carbohydrates and fats as they spent most of their time gathering for carbohydrates from grasses or fruits or they were hunting for days running after a small dear or wild boar.

Our sedentary lifestyles have decoupled the connection between work and food collection. It is possible to use another allegory: salaries today for the most part, are so high that only a fraction of the money earned with physical work is needed to provide for food. Therefore, the affluence of money let us buy more food than we need.

Having such a perspective allows the conclusion that food is an agent-like medicine. We need to know and calculate what our body needs by summing up the energy consumption of our activities and then give the body no more nutrition than it needs.

How food functions in our bodies?

The intake of nutrients must meet the needs of the cells which are dictated by their activity. If there is no energy intake provided by food the metabolic processes will slow down and finally stop—and the organism will die.

So, we can also look at diets that include nutrients instead of excluding them as we urgently need them to guarantee the survival of our cell structures. If we take this point of view we only have to look what food we choose—what medicine we take and what doses of it we need.

If we can educate ourselves to be disciplined in our food preparation and eating it can be the base for a totally new and healthy diet.

Knowing the interaction between diseases and food

We have already discussed the problems which unbalanced diets cause to our health. Even our Western societies are having a high life expectancy, the upside-down age pyramids show that more and more old people have to be supported by the younger ones, but there are hidden factors which should act as a warning sign:

- High absenteeism is registered in our workforces.
- Psychological diseases like depressions are on the rise
- Chronic physical diseases like stress induced serious back and neck pains are reducing productivity.
- The expenditures for chronic diseases are a majority of the health budgets.

Researchers have proven that these problems are partly related to diets.

Certain Cancers, heart diseases and strokes as well as diabetes 2 and obesity were in earlier days said to be caused by genetic issues. Today researchers are getting more and more convinced that all these diseases are created by biological malfunctions.

The nutrients we take in are important factors of this malfunctioning mainly because our diets are not having the necessary balance of nutrients.

We need to know that we can prevent these diseases only if we learn how multiple portions of foods in a diet interact and either disturb or support body functions. IIn all honest, what is a long life good for if there is no quality of life.

I know this is a question which belongs to the medical philosophy, but specifically the ones who lived good and fulfilled lives in their active years are horrified with a low-quality life when they get older.

It is wrong to look at food only as only providing fuel or as a providing agent, which does nothing more than feed the energy we lost through activity.

Modern medicine has a more holistic point of view: They see the digestive, the detoxification and the immune system as an interacting complex system. Was before the immune system only looked at as antibody production in the blood, today we recognize that issues with the digestive system could have influence to the total healthy immunologic function of our body.

Chronic health issues are not coming out of the blue. They are always preceded by declining health of one or more of the body's systems. Finding the underlying causes of malfunctions which lead to a disease is a new approach the functional medicine branch is looking for today.

So far, an introduction to the health impact of food is only a question of a philosophical point of view: Is medicine food or is food medicine?

The first aspect is more of a practical one. In some English-speaking countries there will be the question: *Have you already eaten, or did you already drink your medicine?* There is a described action of consuming something. Like: *Have you already eaten your bread or did you drink your coffee?* We can only speculate if people expressing such sentences see medicine as a food. Is food a medicine? Is a totally different question. Furthermore, there have been discussions on the issue concerning—at what point is food a medicine? Is it a question of the volume and weight? There are voluminous medicines like infusion solutions which are introduced in volumes of more than a liter and there are solid medicines like active carbon to be swallowed to stop diarrhea or absorb poisons in the stomach and the digestive system.

If we can agree that everything which is taken in through the mouth in some way gets metabolized is easy to consent. It is better to conclude, based on our classical understanding of medicine that if taken in too large or too low volumes can be good or bad.

Let us remember Paracelsus: "The **dose** makes the poison."

If we give our body too little of the carbohydrate medicine it will suffer and refuse the service and if we give it too much like the example of the wine, we will destroy vital organs like the liver which, interconnected to the rest of the system, can cause all kinds of diseases like diabetes, cirrhosis or cancer. Today with all our modern diagnostic and laboratory instruments it seems to be easy to measure and check how much of what is good for us.

Recorded human culture is more than 5000 years old. We have good records available from the ancient Egyptians. They already had established a great construction culture. They were brilliant Mathematicians and knew quite a lot about warfare.

However, they had no refined balances or volume measuring instrumentation such as those in use today to measure our food and medicines in doses of milligrams and milliliters.

Mentioning Egypt first is intentional to lead into the first food cultures: The Nile valley is part of the Mediterranean basin and called the cradle of the (Western) Culture. One after another, great cultures were coming and going like the Assyrians, the people living in the Euphrates and Tigris Valley, the Greeks and the Romans and in North Africa the Phoenicians and Moroccans are closely related to the Berbers.

All these cultures had their ups and downs: Partially because they were world powers. Like the Romans, the Greeks developed the earliest democracy and the Egyptians left monuments like the pyramids and the Sphinx. Gone or not, replaced by invaders or intermingled with Germanics or Arabs, one culture has been developed regardless of wars or movements of the borders—the Mediterranean Food Culture.

If you asked the man on the street, if he would know what Mediterranean food culture is; he would immediately know and mention Pizza and Pasta and generally, that is where his knowledge would end. If he is of Jewish or other Mid-Eastern heritage he might know about Falafel or if you meet somebody from Morocco or southern France, couscous might be the answer. A Spaniard might call for paella with real saffron. All are a little right but in general wrong. Mediterranean food is culture.

Over time the origins of the Mediterranean diet got lost. Originally it was identified as bread, wine and olive oil. It was enriched with sheep cheese and vegetables like mushrooms chicory lettuce and leeks. Only little meat and lots of seafood for the people bordering the Mediterranean (Romans could not get enough of it).

Fresh fish was the food of the rich classes which ate it mostly fried in olive oil. The slaves and the poor had bread with olives and olive oil and if they had a good owner or worked in a generous household salted fish and little meat to enrich their diets. Later food from the Germanic neighbors was imported. The Germans brought their hunted, farmed or gathered foods. There are also reports that the Germans had imported the first beers made of the grains in their farms and bartered it with Mediterranean red wines.

But the Romans still mostly stayed with their oil, bread and wine diet. The Germanic trade products were more of an exotic to them. With the monastic orders, the Mediterranean diets were more successful than the Germanics with Evangelization transferring over Roman eating habits.

While the Romans hardly made it with their imperialistic wars over the Rhine River to the east the cuisine made it without costing lives. While bread, oil and wine are parts of the Roman Catholic liturgy some altar boy got first contacts with Mediterranean wine serving the priest in the mass by taking his part and diluted the rest for the diabetic Monsignor.

To the mix of the now Roman/Germanic food came the influence of the Arabs who had, on the Southern beaches of the Mediterranean Sea, developed their own original food cultures. The Muslims now with their siege of a major part of the Spanish Peninsula for nearly 900 years and taught their Christian subservients in a productive and mostly friendly togetherness, how to plant spices, sugar cane spinach eggplant rice and citrus fruits. Rose water, oranges, almonds and lemons became part of the diet of the northern shore Mediterranean area.

After Columbus's detection of the Americas, totally new groups of food entered the Mediterranean basin.

With the silver and gold galleons came the longer lasting riches to Spain: Corn and beans in all colors, potatoes and tomatoes, peppers and chili. The tomato was first considered due to its shining red color as a decorative fruit only and became the signature vegetable of the Mediterranean diet many years later.

So as we can see the Mediterranean diet is nothing static. It has elements from the Egyptian culture to what we know today is a result of a peaceful culture clash between the Romans, Greeks, Germanic tribes on the African shore. At that time the Moroccans, Libyans and Phoenicians and the occupying Arabs in Spain came along with fruits and vegetables brought to Europe after the Americas have been detected.

The Mediterranean diet is mostly identified with vegetables, but vegetables alone do not fill hungry stomachs. Therefore, any report about the Mediterranean wholesome diet would be incomplete without the cereals developed in parallel. Only with them the whole diet makes sense, the various breads, the polenta made of cornmeal, the couscous in France and Morocco, the saffron spiced paella in Spain and not to forget the pasta. Without these cereals the armies, the slaves and the poor could not have been fed and would have revolted because of unsaturated hunger pangs.

The Mediterranean diet is today a worldwide recognized model of food culture.

A diet today only identified as a food consumption method or a doctor prescribed instruction has in his origin Greek word δίαιτα (diaita) the sense of "way of life" or "lifestyle." It reflects a unique mixture of cultures and when we order our pizza today we hardly combine the tomatoes coming originally from Latin America, the olives from Greece or Spain the salami from Italy the Sardines from the African coast and the saffron from Morocco.

It is a simple way of food preparation but it is taking advantage of all points of view of a healthy way of life. It reflects the traditions of many cultures long or midterm gone already and some parts originating from far corners of the world like Latin America.

Here is a citation from the Iranian Journal of Public Health

Tehran University of Medical Sciences

The Mediterranean Diet: A History of Health

Roberta ALTOMARE, Francesco CACCIABAUDO, [...], and Attilio Ignazio LO MONTE

Mediterranean diet: eating behaviors and lifestyles

The discovery of the health benefits of the Mediterranean Diet is attributed to the American scientist Ancel Keys of the University of Minnesota School of Power, which pointed out the correlation between cardiovascular disease and diet for the first time (11). Ancel Keys, in the fifties, was struck by a phenomenon, which could not, at first, provide a full explanation. The poor population of small towns of southern Italy was, against all predictions, much healthier than the wealthy citizens of New York, either of their own relatives who emigrated in earlier decades in the United States. Keys suggested that this depended on food, and tried to validate his original insight, focusing his attention on foods that made up the diet of these populations. Thus, he led the famous "Seven Countries Study" (conducted in Finland, Holland, Italy, United States, Greece, Japan and Yugoslavia), in order to document the relationship between lifestyles, nutrition and cardiovascular disease between different populations, including through cross-sectional studies, being able to prove scientifically the nutritional value of the Mediterranean diet and its contribution to the health of the populations that adopted it (12).

From this study emerged clearly, as the populations that had adopted a diet based on the Mediterranean Diet presented a very low rate of cholesterol in the blood and, consequently, a minimum percentage of coronary heart disease. This was mainly due to the plentiful use of olive oil, bread, pasta, vegetables, herbs, garlic, red onions, and other foods of vegetable origin compared to a rather moderate use of meat (13).

The American nutritionist described the Mediterranean diet in this way: "... homemade minestrone, pasta of all varieties, with tomato sauce and a sprinkling of Parmesan, only occasionally enriched with a few pieces of meat or served with a small fish of the place beans and macaroni ..., so much bread, never removed from the oven more than a few hours before being eaten, and nothing with which spread it, lots of fresh vegetables sprinkled with olive oil, a small portion of meat or fish maybe a couple of times a week and always fresh fruit for dessert"(14).

Many studies have proven that the Mediterranean diet reduces cardiovascular diseases, High density lipoproteins (HDL) are increased and LDL is decreased as well as triglycerides. Going together with a lower Blood pressure and blood glucose.

This not to be construed as direct health medical advice, that only Medical doctors can and are allowed to give—the Mediterranean Diet alone does not work if other risk factors, like smoking, are not reduced and a sedative lifestyle without physical activity is not changed to include regular exercise. The NIH (National Institute of Health) confirmed that moderate physical activity is associated with a decrease in mortality from cardiovascular disease.

Another important citation from the same Article states that: "The relationships between the macronutrient energy answer to those recognized as adequate, i.e. 55–60% carbohydrates of which 80% are complex carbohydrates (bread, pasta, rice), 10–15% of proteins, about 60% are of animal origin (especially white meat, fish) and 25–30% fat (mostly olive oil)."

End of Citation

The Jewel of Mediterranean Diet: Moroccan Food

After covering the Mediterranean diet as a general food philosophy around the Mediterranean basin the special diet of Morocco will get closer attention.

Morocco is located in the Northwestern corner of Africa. Morocco is slightly larger in area than California, and its territory has three different regions. The Northern coast along the Mediterranean Sea is made up of fertile land that rises to elevations of about 8,000 feet (2,400 meters). The Atlas Mountains run between the Atlantic coasts in the southwest to the Mediterranean Sea in the Northeast. Finally, the semiarid area in the south and east known as the Western Sahara connects Morocco with the vast African Sahara Desert.

Morocco faces a problem with Desertification. This is a process where fertile land becomes unfertile and desert-like. Desertification may be caused by forces of nature, such as lack of rainfall or drought. In the Northwest, agriculture in Morocco thrives. Except in years when there is severe drought, Moroccan farmers are able to supply the country with enough food.

Moroccan diet history: Nomads called Berbers were the first inhabitants of Morocco over two thousand years ago. They used local ingredients, such as olives, figs, and dates, to prepare lamb and poultry stews. Over time, traders and conquering nations introduced new food customs. Among them were the Phoenicians, Carthaginians, and Romans. However, the strongest influence on native cooking was the Arab invasion in the seventh century A.D.

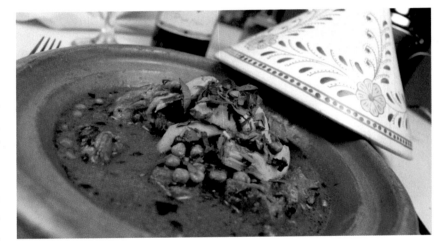

The Arabs brought with them new breads and other foods made from grains. They introduced spices including cinnamon, ginger, saffron, cumin, and caraway. They also introduced sweet-and-sour cooking, which they had learned from the Persians. Moors from Andalusia in southern Spain also influenced Moroccan cooking. In modern times, the French and the British made contributions to Moroccan cuisine.

Morocco, unlike most other African countries, produces all the food it needs to feed its people. Its many home-grown fruits and vegetables include oranges, melons, tomatoes, sweet and hot peppers, and potatoes. Five more native products that are especially important in Moroccan cooking are lemons, olives, figs, dates, and almonds. Located on the coast of the Mediterranean Sea, the country is rich in fish and seafood. Beef is not plentiful, so meals are usually built around lamb or poultry.

Flat, round Moroccan bread is eaten at every meal. The Moroccan national dish is lamb or poultry stew. Other common ingredients may include almonds, hard-boiled eggs, prunes, lemons, tomatoes, and other vegetables. The Tajine, like other Moroccan dishes, is known for its distinctive flavoring, which comes from spices including saffron, cumin, coriander, cinnamon, ginger, and ground red pepper. The tajine's name is taken from the distinctive earthenware dish with a cone-shaped top in which it is cooked and served. Another Moroccan staple is couscous, made from fine grains of a wheat product called semolina. It is served many different ways, with vegetables, meat, or seafood.

Sweets have very important role in the Moroccan diet. Every household has a supply of homemade sweet desserts made from almonds, honey, and other ingredients. Mint tea is served with every meal in Morocco. It is sweetened while it is still in the pot.

Morocco, being a predominantly Muslim country has religious dietary restrictions that prohibit the consumption of pork and alcohol. During the holy season of Ramadan, when Muslims fast during the day, a thick soup called harira is served at night. A bowl of harira, which is made with beans and lamb, is served with fresh dates. It is served both at home and in cafes. For the holiday Eid al-Fitr, which marks the end of Ramadan, a holiday feast is prepared. A popular dish at this feast is bisteeya, made with pigeon meat wrapped in pastry dough. More than 100 layers of pastry dough may be used in the preparation of this dish.

The Muslim feast day of Eid el Kebir takes place seventy days after Ramadan. For this holiday, a sheep is roasted on a spit and served whole at the table. Each person cuts off a piece and dips it into a dish of cumin. Rich date bars called mescouta are a popular dessert on many festive occasions.

Moroccans eat their meals at low round tables, sitting on cushions on the floor. They eat with their hands instead of silverware, using the thumb and first two fingers of their right hands. They also use pieces of bread to soak up sauces and carry food to the mouth. Small warmed, damp towels are passed around before the meal to make sure everyone's hands are clean. Most meals consist of a single main dish, often a stew, a couscous dish, or a hearty soup. It is served with bread, salad, cold vegetables, and couscous or rice on the side. A typical breakfast might include beyssara (dried fava beans stewed with cumin and paprika), beghrir (pancakes), and bread. Two breakfast favorites that may sound exotic to Westerners are lambs' heads and calves' feet.

Although Moroccans love sweets, they are usually saved for special occasions. With everyday meals, the most common dessert is fresh fruit. The sweetened mint tea that comes with every meal is served a special way. It is brewed in a silver teapot and served in small glasses. When the tea is poured, the pot is held high above the glasses to let air mix with the tea. Tea is served not only at home but also in public places. In stores, merchants often offer tea to their customers.

Morocco is famous for the wide range of delicious foods sold by its many street vendors. These include soup, shish kebab, roasted chickpeas, and salads. Both full meals and light snacks are sold. A favorite purchase is sugared doughnuts tied together on a string to carry home.

Conclusion

So far you have been introduced to Moroccan food. We tried to build a correlation of general diets to the functions of food in our body. We hypothesized on food is a medicine and we studied the development of the food culture in the Mediterranean basin.

The final more specific study is covering the Moroccan diet—a combination of food culture from the Mediterranean basin.

Morocco adds to the already rich Mediterranean food culture a development of a diet going far back to the Berbers the oldest inhabitants of this North West African country with a partial coastline at the Mediterranean Sea.

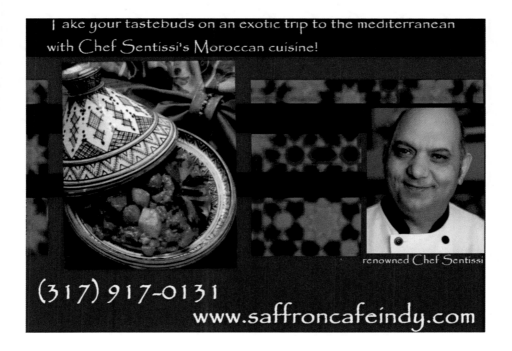

Introduction

This section of recipes presents many different ways to incorporate fresh, wholesome, nutritious and delicious food into the diet as well as instructions on consuming all meals holistically. It means a change of habits in eating. A lifelong eating habit cannot be changed just by reading a different rule. It needs constant training to consider food intake as an essential part of the behavior not filling the stomach to get rid of the hunger which shows frequently and punctually before breakfast, lunch and dinner or even snack times in between. These frequencies and punctuality alone show that the change of habits will not be an easy one.

Eating any type of meal needs to be considered to integrate nourishment as a part of life like working, resting, or sleeping. Only with such strict a kind of approach will allow healing by eating can begin.

Eating holistically permits detoxification of the body naturally. It creates more energy and promotes a satiated feeling for a longer time with a clear mind and stable moods. After feeling so good eating habits change to the positive and the spiral of making healthier food choices starts to turn in the right direction.

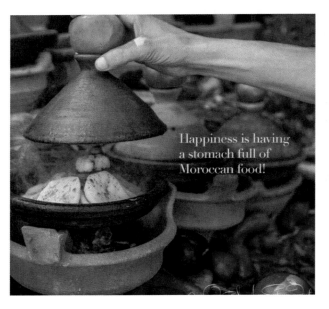

Happiness is having a stomach full of Moroccan food!

The key to unlock the door to a life of vitality and wellness is now at hand, the journey to optimal health and wellness can start from here.

This journey begins in the mind with the ingredients chosen carefully. A commitment from preparation to consumption is the first step to get the most out of the food to be eaten. It can be seen as the first training step too.

The basis of this philosophy is that food can be seen as medicine and capable not only of maintaining the health, but has a potential to improve it. By eating not only healthy, but holistically and constantly considering not just what is eaten, but how the nutrients are consumed we can improve the quality of life and will experience improvement.

The recognition that food as medicine is gaining momentum and power. This is not to discount the achievements of modern medicine, but a call to return to simple eating. Forgetting the misconceptions that nourishing the body properly can be done by quickly passing through a drive-in restaurant—a resurgence to appreciate the importance of food and respecting the time which needs to be taken for a meal.

People who prepare their own meals are known they take their time to enjoy in preparation and eating reap benefits just from the process of lovingly creating their meals and being grateful for every bite they prepared for their family and themselves.

Digestion is an important part of the nourishment process. Planning the diet for a good digestion is part of providing for healthy eating.

Manufactured foods and additives disturb our bodies and complicate digestion. This contributes to unnatural weight gain, disease, and common maladies that plague us throughout the day. Our bodies are biologically suited over Millenniums for processing natural food. It must be considered that manufactured foods are a result of affluence. The majority of Western societies have only been bombarded with processed foods since the early fifties. Our parents and grandparents baked their own breads, made their noodles and butchered their home raised cattle, fish and chicken and brewed their own beer, wine and coffee surrogate out of barley.

In order to create a diet that is body friendly and natural some preferences and likings have to be eliminated. Namely nutrients that disagree with the digestion. The best way to go is to eliminate some diets. By eating a wide range of foods and carefully keeping records of the results on what works best with the body, one not only learns to listen to the body, but also learns what foods are best.

This process brings the individual eating habits in tune with the body and closer to a holistic approach to eating. The body is the most natural marker of what is good and what is bad an excellent indicator on how to customize a diet.

Change is seldom easy. It may take time to find, prepare, and eat healthy every day, especially in the phase of transition. There will also be a detoxification period where the body still craves for the unhealthy ingredients of the previous old diet. That is okay. Patience is required with the change of personal habits. It may not be easy, but changing a diet and the mind respecting the powerful natural force of food will be worth the effort.

Chapter 7: Making it All Work Together

You know that you are different from everyone else because of your DNA and because of your background. That doesn't mean that you cannot benefit from the basic principles of eating whole foods and integrating various ingredients into your diet.

Dr. Andrew Weil has talked about whole mill products versus processed dairy and how it's possible to reduce the amount of inflammation in the body by learning what to eat. He uses a balance of caloric intake, carbohydrates, fat, protein, fiber, phytonutrients, vitamins and minerals and other dietary supplements to establish what a nutritious plate should be. The "Anti-inflammatory Diet" that he has created is not actually a diet but a lifestyle change. It focuses on being informed about food choices, which is what this eBook is all about – making healthy decisions in terms of what you eat.

My program is simple because it emphasizes some of the nutrient-dense animal foods that are pasteurized and grain fed but also a large amount of fruits, vegetables, and healthy dietary fats. Continual detoxification of the body is important to ensure the systems operate properly and that the body is running at the highest possible level.

I often quote Hippocrates when talking about food – "Let thy food be thy medicine and let they medicine be thy food". These are truly words to live by and is further evidence of the holistic approach that needs to be taken when you talk about the foods you need to eat in order to be a healthier person.

There are ways that you can bring the information that you have learned throughout this book together. You can decide to get a health coach, make a dinner reservation at the Saffron Café, or simply follow some of the recipes that are listed below.

My recipes are packed with saffron, garlic, and other anti-inflammatory ingredients. They are rich with vitamins, nutrients, and antioxidants, which means that each forkful is loaded with goodness and will help you in one way or another. More importantly, the food tastes good!

Happy cooking!

Conclusion

At the end of the day, you want to be sure that you eat food that is good for you. What is good for **you** may not be good for someone else, so you have to listen to the cues that your body gives you. There are some ingredients that are universally good for everyone, so incorporating them into your diet is always a good thing.

The more you know about the ingredients that you cook with and that are found in your favorite foods, the easier it will be to make educated decisions about what you put in your body.

Saffron is a great ingredient that does a lot of good things for the body. When combined with other great ingredients, you have a recipe for success throughout the year. Whether you follow the recipes in this book or you come to visit the Saffron Café for dinner or for cooking lessons, you will learn the benefits of using this ingredient – and how you can manipulate the ingredient to match the types of foods that you want to eat.

Moroccan Recipes for Holistic Living

Good food doesn't just fill your belly, it nourishes you, your body and your soul. In a world of highly-processed fast food and cuisines that lean heavily on meats and fats to provide substance and flavor, much of what you put into your body may satisfy the tongue at the expense of your health. Both in running our restaurants and writing this book, we aimed to change that by diving deep into a healthy, exotic, and downright delectable culinary tradition: Moroccan Mediterranean cuisine.

Moroccan food isn't just good for you, it's exciting. It explores the balance of bold spices and bright, fresh vegetables bursting with flavor as well as vitamins and antioxidants. It never leaves vegetarians or vegans feeling left out when there are show-stopping options like harira lentil and tomato soup or the rich zaalouk eggplant salad, a perfect accompaniment to a cup of steaming tea and a slice of crusty bread. Meat-eaters will find their meals taken to a new level with the exquisite spices of kafta-prepared meats, where every bite brings a delightful interplay of flavors.

Whether it's the fresh herbs, the sunny taste of olive oil, or the masterful use of vegetables either as a side or as a worthy dish in their own right, Moroccan Mediterranean food has a kind of health you can taste and feel from your tongue to your satisfied stomach. Without trans fats, ingredients of dubious repute, or heavily-processed additives, you'll find yourself eating meals that are among the most wholesome you can prepare.

As you go through the recipes in this book, we hope you'll gain a new appreciation for what can be done with fresh ingredients, whole foods, and a good dose of North African tradition.

Introduction to Moroccan Cuisine:

Colorful, spicy, sweet and scented – that just about sums up Moroccan food! Wherever you go in Morocco a heady aroma of cinnamon, ginger, turmeric, cumin and coriander (cilantro) wafts through the streets drawing you in to the busy food stalls and restaurants selling deliciously tempting snacks and dishes. From the inspired fruity salads spiked with chilies and tangy olives to the syrupy, buttery tajines topped with preserved lemon and the light grains of fluffy couscous combined with saffron, nuts and fresh herbs, there an amazing variety of dishes, all with their unique health benefits.

Seasoned by the flavor of Moroccan culture, the country's cuisine is a fascinating reflection of the history of a country whose invaders, such as the ancient Phoenicians and Romans, have come and gone, each leaving a stamp on the culinary landscape. Starting around 1100BC, the culinary history includes the indigenous Berber population, which inhabited the inland fertile plains and the harsh mountainous terrain where they lived on honey, beans, lentils and wheat and began the lifelong tradition of tajine cooking and couscous; the nomadic Bedouins from the desert who brought dates, milk and grains; the Moors, expelled from Spain relied heavily on olives and olive oil and brought with them the Andalusian flavors of paprika and herbs; the Sephardic Jews with their preserving techniques employing salt. The Arabs who introduced the sophisticated cuisine from the Middle East along with Islamic culinary restrictions; slaves from central Africa with their tribal culinary secrets; the Ottoman influence of kebabs and pastry making; and the French, who left a legacy of wine-making, café culture, and general culinary finesse.

To absorb the delights and diversity of Morocco's cuisine it is worth visiting the markets of the larger cities such as Marrakech and Fez where the labyrinthine souks are the centers of all social and culinary activity. Among the make-shift barber's shops and stalls, you can find vendors selling cones of raw sugar, shampoo stones, dried lizards and snake skins, and the butchered carcasses of cows and sheep. Mini emporiums displaying carpets, leather goods, clothing, jewelry and pottery abound. There is much to buy and admire. In the culinary realm, you can find utensils carved from lemon wood and juniper bark, traditional clay tajines, dried herbs and spices, fleshy olives of every color and size; tiny preserved lemons, and argan oil, the precious pressing of the roasted kernels of the argan nut which is extracted from the excretions of the goats that climb the stout, thorny trees!

Generally, Moroccan meals begin with a selection of cold salads and small dishes, such as bowls of fava bean salad, marinated carrot salad, slices of tiny spicy *merguez* (cured sausage), pickled vegetables, stuffed pastries, and mini meat balls. These dishes are designed to whet the appetite for the ensuing soup or tajine, followed by grilled or roasted meat, and finally a mound of couscous. Fresh fruit usually completes the meal or, on occasion, a sweet milk pudding or pastry scented with rose or orange blossom water. Once everything has been cleared away, glasses of steaming mint tea will be served to aid the digestion while you sit back and reflect on all the wonderful dishes you have consumed!

Please enjoy discovering the delights and health benefits of these dishes inspired by traditional Moroccan cooking!

Brief Overview of Moroccan History:

The area of modern Morocco has been inhabited since Neolithic times, at least 8000 BC, as attested by signs of the ancient Capsian culture (the precursors of the Berber people), in a time when the Maghreb (or region of Berber cultural prevalence) was less arid than it is today. Many experts believe the *Amazigh* language, commonly referred to as Berber, probably arrived at roughly the same time as agriculture, and was adopted by the existing population and the immigrants that brought it.

Modern genetic analyses have confirmed that various populations have contributed to the present-day population of Morocco, including (and in addition to the main Berber and Arab groups) Jews, sub-Saharan Africans, and Western Europeans of the Mediterranean cultural sphere. The Berbers, often referred to in modern ethnic activist circles as "Amazigh" are more commonly known as "Berber" or by their regional ethnic identity, such as Chleuh. In the classical period, Morocco was known as Mauretania, although this should not be confused with the modern country of Mauritania.

North Africa and Morocco were slowly drawn into the wider emerging Mediterranean world by Phoenician trading colonies and settlements in the late Classical period. The Phoenicians explored this corner of Africa around 1000 B.C.E. and found the area away from the coast to be inhabited by people they called barbaroi (meaning "not our people"), which later became known as the Berbers. The Berbers may have had links with the Celts, Basques, or tribes from the Lebanon. Around 150 B.C.E., the Romans added this part of the North African coast to their empire but did not generally disturb the Berbers, who were largely further inland and in the mountains. The 7th century C.E. saw Arab armies spread across northern Africa and into Morocco. They didn't stop there though. They joined with the Berbers and later invaded most of Spain, where they had a presence for around 800 years.

In 788, a descendant of the Prophet Mohammed, named Moulay Idriss, was proclaimed king by the Berber tribes. Moulay Idriss quickly became a powerful and influential figure, but was murdered by a rival. The village which is the location of his tomb is now called Moulay Idriss and is one of the most sacred shrines in Morocco. The son of Moulay Idriss, Moulay Idriss II, took over and founded the present city of Fez, the capital for a time afterwards. After his death in 828, power was split between his several sons, resulting in a weakness of leadership.

In the mid-11th century, an army of strict Muslims, the mainly Berber Almoravids, moved out from their fortified monastery in the desert to the south and conquered southern Morocco, destroying musical instruments, drinking places, and other establishments they deemed to be irreverent as they went. The Almoravids eventually captured Fez, after founding their own capital at Marrakesh and later had influence in Spain as well.

Later, in the mid-12th century, another fanatic group, the Almohads, moved from their fortified monastery in the Atlas Mountains to take control of all of North Africa and much of Spain. Eventually, the Almohads were weakened by infighting. In the mid-13th century, the Beni Merin Berber tribe took control. The Merinids were more materialistic than their predecessors, and under their rule many masterpieces of architecture were built, including the Alhambra at Granada, Spain.

After the Christians eventually pushed the Moors (Arabs and Berbers) out of Spain, the Spanish and Portuguese invaded the Moroccan coastline (Spain still holds control of Ceuta and Melilla on the north Moroccan coast to this day). This encouraged the Saadi Arab tribe from the Draa valley to move north and eventually take control during the mid to late 16th century, bringing King Ahmed el Mansour to power. The Saadians lavished much wealth on Marrakesh.

After King Ahmed's death in the early 17th century, the Saadian's power fell apart and allowed the Alaouites to take control under Sultan Moulay Ismail. In fact, the Alaouites were invited by the people of Fez to restore order to the country. Ismail was believed to be cruel and ruthless but was also a leader and restored order. The Alaouites kept control for over two centuries but during the 19th century, Morocco fell increasingly under France's sphere of influence (Europe had been colonizing Africa and the French had taken control of Morocco's neighbor, Algiers).

In 1912. Morocco became a Franco-Spanish protectorate but with an Alaouite sultan, chosen by the French. The French controlled the central and southern areas while the Spanish controlled north. Tangiers was the main international zone and Rabat the capital at the time. During this time, the Franco-Spanish influence resulted in numerous roads, railways, and schools being built and many new towns were built beside the old.

The Second World War weakened the position of the French and there was a surge of a strong movement for Moroccan independence. To control this, the French exiled the sultan Mohamad V to Corsica, but only succeeded in strengthening the independence movement. Eventually the French had to bring Mohamed V back and he became king in 1956, when independence was declared.

King Mohamed V died suddenly and unexpectedly in 1961 and was succeeded by his son, Hassan II, who introduced a Social, Democratic and Constitutional monarchy, with elections for the parliament every 6 years but power remaining with the king. The present king, Mohamad VI, succeeded king Hassan II on his death in 1999, has continued his father's progressive reforms in areas such as health, education, and economics. Morocco is modernizing but also retaining its unique traditions and culture.

Signature Spices and Ingredients in Moroccan Cuisine

Basil

Basil is a tender low-growing herb prominently featured in Mediterranean cuisine. The leaves and stems plant tastes somewhat like anise, with a strong, pungent, sweet smell. Scientific studies have established that compounds in basil oil have potent antioxidant hence anti-aging, anti-cancer, anti-viral, and anti-microbial properties.

Bay Laurel

Also known as bay leaf, this herb is often used to flavor soups, stews, braises and pates in Mediterranean Cuisine. It is an antioxidant, and has analgesic and anti-inflammatory properties.

Cloves

Cloves have historically been used throughout the world to enhance the presentation and flavor of rice, stews, Broths, and Meats. Cloves are also a key ingredient in making certain types of tea. In certain traditional medicine practices, cloves have been used as a prominent ingredient in emergency medicine. Its pain reduction properties can help skin disorders and burns, and also relieves stomach pain and sensitivity.

Coriander

Also known as cilantro, this herb is a soft, hairless plant. It is most commonly used to add a citrus-like overtone to dishes. Since diminishes their flavor quickly, coriander leaves are often used raw or added to the dish right before serving.

Cumin

Cumin is thought to be the second most popular spice in the world today after black pepper. It's distinctive flavor and strong warm aroma is due to its essential oil content that draws the natural sweetness from a dish. Cumin is classified as a stimulant, a carminative (decreasing or preventing the formulation of gas in the digestive system) and an anti-microbial agent.

Curry Powder

Curry powder is a mixture of spices of widely varying composition that is a classic in Mediterranean cuisine. It was largely popularized during the nineteenth and twentieth centuries through the mass exportation of the condiment to the Western table throughout Europe as well as North and South America.

Dill

Made from fresh and dried dill leaves, this herb's fern-like leaves are aromatic and serve a variety of spicing purposes in many dishes.

Fennel Seed

Dried fennel seed is an aromatic, anise-flavored spice used in many Moroccan side dishes, salads, and pasta. In traditional medicine, Fennel has a widespread use varying from vision improvement to relieving chronic coughing

Ginger

Ginger is a very popular spice used to prepare chicken, vegetables and curries. Young ginger rhizomes are juicy and fleshy with a very mild taste. Ginger has been classified as a stimulant and a carminative, commonly used to treat arthritis and heart disease. More recently, ginger has been employed to disguise the taste of medicine. It is also an effective aid in digestion and has antimicrobial properties

Ras Hanout

Ras el hanout is a popular blend of herbs and spices that is used across the Middle East and North Africa. The name means "head of the shop" in Arabic, and refers to a mixture of the best spices a seller has to offer. While there is no definitive set combined spices, I have my own secret combination of over 12 herbs and spices

Oregano

Oregano is often used in tomato sauces, with fried vegetables, and grilled meat. Together with basil, it contributes much to the distinctive character of many Moroccan dishes. It has an aromatic, warm and slightly bitter taste that varies in intensity. Oregano is high in antioxidant activity, demonstrating useful characteristics in relieving stomach and respiratory ailments.

Paprika

Paprika is used as an ingredient in a broad variety of dishes throughout the world. Paprika is principally used to season the color in rice, stews and soups. The herb is rich in Vitamin C and antioxidants.

Black Pepper

Used since nearly 2000 BC, black pepper is one of the most common spices in Mediterranean and various international cuisines.

Rosemary

The fresh and dried leaves are frequently used in traditional Mediterranean cuisine. They have a bitter, astringent taste which compliments a wide variety of foods. Rosemary is extremely high in iron calcium and Vitamin B6. Rosemary also contains camosic acid, which lowers the risk of strokes and neurodegenerative diseases like Alzheimer's and ALS.

Sesame Seeds

Sesame seed is grown primarily for its oil-rich seeds that come in a variety of colors and have many different culinary uses. They are added to bread, baked into crackers or roasted in desserts. The seeds are rich in manganese, copper, calcium and other vitamins and are commonly used as an antioxidant and associated with lowering blood cholesterol.

Tarragon

Tarragon compliments certain types of fish, meat, soups and stews quite well, and is often used in tomato and egg dishes. Its slightly bittersweet aroma adds distinctive flavor to sauces. It is also known to help fight off fatigue and calm the nerves.

Thyme

Thyme is often used to flavor meats, soups and stews. It has a particular affinity to, and is often used as a primary flavor with lamb, tomatoes and eggs. Thyme, while flavorful, does not overpower a dish when used in moderation and blends well with other herbs and spices. This herb contains thymol, an antiseptic commonly used in mouthwash and medicated bandages.

Turmeric

Tumeric is sometimes used to impart a rich, custard-like yellow color to savory dishes and has found application in nearly every spectrum of food production. While commonly used as an antiseptic for cuts, burns, and bruises, this spice can also support nerve growth, aids in treating depression, and decreases the risk of cancer.

Saffron

Saffron is a very costly spice, used to flavor and color food. The spice is actually the dried stigma (tiny threadlike strands) of the Crocus Sativus Linneaus, a member of the iris family. The flower's stigma accepts the pollen that is produced by the stamen, which becomes the seeds of the next generation. Each stigma is very small, and tens of thousands of individual strands go into a single ounce of the spice. Since the stigmas are hand-plucked from the individual flowers, saffron's high cost becomes more understandable. Saffron is indeed the most expensive spice in the world.

Saffron originated in the Middle East, but is now also associated with Greek, Indian and Spanish cuisines. Fortunately, a very little saffron goes a long way — it is a spice to be added one thread at a time. Just a thread or two can flavor and color an entire pot of rice. The flavor is distinctive and pungent. Most 'saffron rice' mixes commercially available actually use a substitute which dyes the rice the distinctive yellow but which does not impart the flavor of true saffron.

For therapeutic purposes, saffron it is considered an excellent stomach ailment and an antispasmodic (relieving muscle cramps and spasms), and helps in digestion and increasing appetite.

It is also provides relief of renal colic, reduces stomachaches and relieves tension. During recent years, it was used as a drug for flu-like infections, depression and as a sedative for its essential oils. It is also considered that in small quantities it regulates menstruation and helps conception. In the pharmaceutical industry, 125 grams of pure saffron essence is enough for making 300 million sedative tablets.

Saffron is given to reduce fevers, cramps and enlarged livers, to calm nerves. In the Western world it is used primarily as a spice. We are now discovering the use of Saffron as a health tonic, which naturally does not have side effects. About 50 mg of Saffron dissolved in a glass of 200ml milk and a spoonful of sugar makes a very tasty drink, which is also a health tonic. Regular intake of this tonic every day for a period of time enables the body to build resistance against many common diseases such as Asthma, Common colds claim Ayurvedic Practitioners. Beware not to expect it to act as a magic potion because it is essential to have a regular intake for it to be effective.

APPETIZERS

Zaalouk

Traditional Moroccan Eggplant Spread

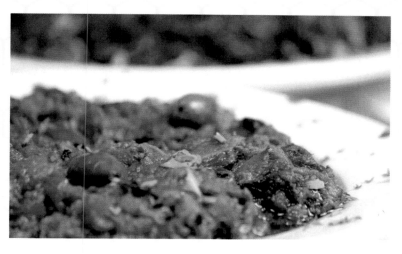

3 large eggplants, peeled and sliced

¼ cup extra-virgin olive oil

Salt, to taste

4 tomatoes, diced

2 onions, peeled and thinly sliced

2 tablespoons cumin

2 tablespoons paprika

Parsley, to taste

Cilantro, to taste

Fresh ground black pepper, to taste

Preheat oven to 350 degrees. Place sliced eggplant onto baking sheet with extra-virgin olive oil and salt. Cook in 350-degree oven until eggplant becomes soft, about 15 minutes.

To a large saucepan, add onions, tomatoes, with the parsley, cilantro, cumin, and paprika to taste. Cook for 15 minutes, stirring occasionally.

Remove the eggplant from the oven and chop into small pieces. Add the eggplant to the saucepan with the onions, tomatoes and seasonings. Add salt and pepper to taste.

Serve with freshly warmed pita bread.

Zucchini Spread

Zaalouk with Zucchini

Zaalouk is a savory spread traditionally made from roasted eggplant. However, Zaalouk can be made from a variety of other roasted vegetables as well. Have fun experimenting with a variety of vegetables and spices. Zaalouk is often served with fresh bread, but to keep it gluten free, it can also be served with rice, bulgar, quinoa, or any other grain. It can also be spread on sliced cucumbers or carrots.

2 large zucchinis

3 tablespoons of vegetable oil

¾ teaspoon of kosher salt

¼ cup of olive oil

2 cups of diced onions

1 cup of fresh tomatoes, diced

3 tablespoons of garlic puree

3 tablespoons of parsley, chopped

3 tablespoons of cilantro, chopped

1 ½ teaspoon of kosher salt

1 tablespoon of cumin

1 tablespoon of paprika

Hummus

6 (15 oz.) can chickpeas, in brine

4 oz. extra virgin olive oil

4 oz. garlic puree

6 oz. tahini

4 oz. cumin

2 tomatoes, diced

Parsley chopped

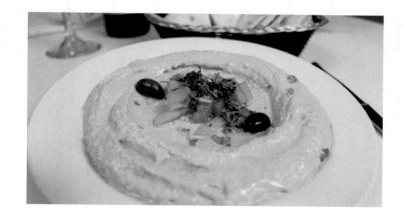

Serve with toasted pita bread

1. Combine all ingredients, minus the tomatoes and parsley, into a large bowl and mix well.

2. Puree in batches. Stir to ensure hummus is mixed well.

3. Serve on plate, drizzle with extra virgin olive oil and garnish with 2 oz. diced tomatoes and chopped parsley. Serve with toasted pita bread.

Bakoula

Traditional Moroccan Spinach Spread

2 lb. box chopped spinach, thawed and drained

¼ cup extra-virgin olive oil

Kosher salt, to taste

4 tomatoes, diced

2 onions, peeled and diced

2 tablespoons cumin

2 tablespoons paprika

Parsley, to taste

Cilantro, to taste

Fresh ground black pepper, to taste

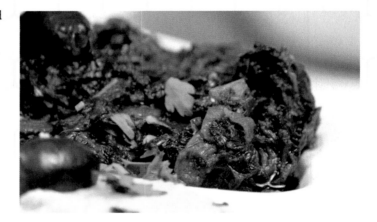

1. In a large saucepan, add the olive oil, onions, tomatoes, parsley and cilantro, to taste, cumin and paprika. Cook for 15 minutes, stirring occasionally.
2. Add the spinach to the saucepan with the onions, tomatoes and seasonings. Add salt and pepper, to taste.
3. Serve with freshly warmed pita bread.

Kale Spread

Bakoula with Kale

Bakoula is a spread traditionally made from chopped spinach, heavily seasoned and exciting. However, bakoula can be made from any sort of leafy green. This recipe uses kale, one of nature's superfoods, rich in iron and vitamin C. Try experimenting with a variety of greens and seasonings. Collards, chard, turnip or beet tops, or dandelion greens are just some of the options you could use. Bakoula is great served with fresh bread, but can also be served alongside any type of delicious grain. It is also delicious accompanied by feta cheese cubes and Kalamata olives.

2 bunches of kale (preferably organic), cleaned and stems removed

3 tablespoons of coconut oil

1 ½ cups of diced onions

¾ cups of diced tomatoes

3 tablespoons of garlic puree

3 tablespoons of parsley, chopped

3 tablespoons of basil, chopped

1 ½ teaspoon of kosher salt

1 tablespoon of cumin

1 tablespoon of paprika

1. Combine all of the ingredients except for the kale in a large pot.
2. Cook over medium heat until tomatoes and onions are very soft (15-20 minutes).
3. Chop the kale into bite sized pieces, add to the pot, and cook for an additional 15 minutes, or until the kale has turned a very dark green.

Taktouka De Meknes

2 char-grilled Bell-red Pepper diced

2 char-grilled Tomatoes Diced

2oz Chopped Parsley

2oz Chopped Cilantro

1 tsp Preserved Lemon Diced fine

Add Charmoula to your taste

Combine all ingredients in mixing Bowl

SALADS

Green Goodness

The best recipe for salads is to be creative combining raw green foods in a salad bowl, add dressing recipes from page 86.

When it comes to superfoods, few readily available products provide us with more nutrients than leafy greens such as spinach, kale and broccoli. Green vegetables give an extra boost to your heart-health as they are high in carotenoids, which act as antioxidants and free your body of potentially harmful compounds.

They're also high in fiber and contain loads of vitamins and minerals. Kale also has some omega-3 fatty acids.

They're especially good for those seeking to maintain nutritional balance whilst following a plant-based or vegan diet, as the nutrient-dense foods such as spinach and kale keep you satiated for longer as they take longer to digest, and provide your body with the nutrition it needs. They're also full of fiber and help to regulate blood sugar levels!

You can't go wrong with including more of these superfoods into your diet!

Green fruits and vegetables contain varying amounts of potent phytochemicals such as lutein and indoles. Benefits include a lower risk of some cancers, improved eye health, rejuvenated musculature and bone, and strong teeth. Stock up on these healthy green foods:

Broccoli – High in calcium and iron, this veggie has been linked to stronger teeth, bones, and muscles, and a decreased risk of cancer.

Spinach – This leafy green is high in antioxidants and vitamin K, which helps strength bones.

Kiwi – Kiwi is high in folate, vitamin E, and glutathione, which all help decrease the risk of heart disease and promote optimal overall health.

Other Green Foods:

Other healthy green foods include avocados, green apples, green grapes, honeydew, limes, pears, artichokes, arugula, asparagus, broccoflower, broccoli rabe, Brussels sprouts, Chinese cabbage, green beans, green cabbage, celery, chayote squash, cucumbers, endives, leafy greens, leeks, lettuce, green onions, green peppers, peas, snow peas, sugar snap peas, watercress, and zucchini.

Orange Avocado Salad

Makes approximately 2-3 servings.

1 large navel orange, peeled and cut into 6 wedges

1 avocado, peeled and cut into 6 wedges

1/2 diced white onion

1/2 cup peeled cucumber, diced

1/2 cup Kalamata olives

Salt, to taste

1/4 cup fresh cilantro, finely diced

2 tbsp. Paprika

1 tsp cinnamon

1 tbsp. Harissa, or to taste

1-2 tsp olive oil

I/2 lemon

Preparation:

In a large salad bowl combine lemon juice, harissa, paprika, cinnamon and salt with Kalamata olives, onion, cucumber and orange sections.

Then carefully fold the avocado wedges into the mixture as well.

On a large plate place each orange section alternating with each avocado wedge in a circle, but leaving an open space in the middle of the circle on the plate.

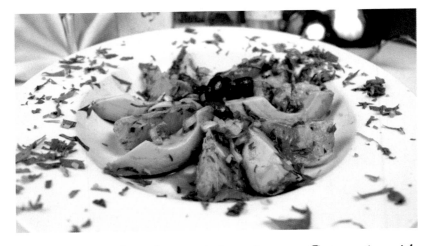

In this remaining central space use a spatula or spoon to place the remaining mixture... Get creative with your plate!

Moroccan Chicken Salad

4 chicken breasts

3 cups of water

1 tablespoon of extra virgin olive oil (can substitute for vegetable oil)

1/3 cup of mayonnaise

½ teaspoon of paprika

½ teaspoon of cumin

½ teaspoon of ginger

Pinch of kosher salt

1/3 cup of raisins

¼ cup of green onions, finely diced

¼ cup of fresh basil

1. In a large pot, bring the water to a boil, adding oil and a pinch of salt.
2. Add chicken and boil until thoroughly cooked, but still tender.
3. Let chicken cool to room temperature, then dice into small cubes
4. Combine chicken, mayonnaise, spices, salt, raisins, green onions, and basil in a large mixing bowl. Mix thoroughly.
5. Enjoy on a sandwich or by itself.

Fresh Mozzarella Salad

Family serving:

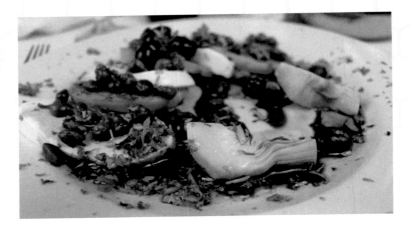

3 fresh tomatoes

1 lb. fresh mozzarella, sliced

3 cups chopped fresh greens: spinach, arugula, and romaine

1/2 cup fresh basil, chopped

4 tbsps. Kalamata olives, diced

3 tbsps. lemon capers

1 lemon, squeezed

3 tbsps. balsamic vinegar

Pinch Kosher salt, to taste

Toss all ingredients together in a large salad bowl.

SOUPS

Harrira Soup

Vegetarian Soup with Saffron Rice, Chick Peas, and Moroccan Spices and Seasonings

6 cups of water

3 tablespoons finely ground celery

2 large onions, diced

3 large tomatoes, finely diced

I cup of cilantro, finely chopped

¼ cup of parsley, finely chopped

1 teaspoon of salt

2 tablespoons of ginger powder

Pinch of freshly ground black pepper

3 tablespoons of butter

1 cup of chick peas

1/2 cup of Basmati rice

Pinch of saffron

1. In a large pot, bring the water to a boil
2. Add celery
3. Add the rice
4. Add the spices and let the mixture simmer for roughly half an hour.
5. Stir frequently
6. Simmer for 10 minutes.
7. Add the chick peas

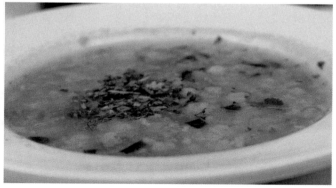

8. Simmer for an additional 3-5 minutes- take care to make sure the rice and chick peas retain their firmness.
9. Harried soup traditionally served in the breakfast or light diner with boiled eggs, dates, and whole grain bread.

Bissara

Traditional Moroccan Fava Bean Soup

2 cups of dried fava beans, soaked in water overnight

2 tablespoons vegetable oil

2 tablespoons pure garlic

1 tsp salt

1 tsp cumin

1tsp paprika (optional)

Water

1. Drain dried fava beans from water. Peel them and rinse well.
2. Place dried fava beans, garlic, oil, spices and water, then cover the soup pan and cook covered on medium heat for an hour or until the fava beans are soft and well-cooked.
3. Mash the beans with a wooden spoon or place them in a processor until the mixture is smooth
4. Return the mashed beans to the cooker and simmer over low heat until the soup becomes thick.
5. Serve the soup in bowls with a drizzle of olive oil, cumin and paprika (optional) on top.

This soup is known as a popular remedy for lung dysfunctions.

Health benefit of beans—high in protein.

Moroccan Lentil Soup

Lentils are a healthy, hearty, and nutritious staple in Middle Eastern and Moroccan cuisine. They are packed with protein and vitamins, as well as being economical and delicious!

1. Drain the soaking water from the lentils and rinse them well.
2. Combine all of the ingredients except for the lentils and butter in a large stock pot.
3. When the soup comes to a boil, add the lentils.
4. Reduce to medium-low heat and simmer for 45 minutes to an hour, until Lentils are soft and tender
5. Remove from heat and add the Butter, stirring gently. If you wish to keep the soup vegan, simply omit the Butter. Can be served with a drizzle of Olive Oil and a light sprinkle of Cayenne Pepper if you like.

Lentils are high in Iron.

Shorba

1 lb. lamb loin chops or beef stew meat

2 onions, finely minced

3 tomatoes, peeled seeded, then crushed

3 carrots, thinly sliced

2 celery stalks, thinly sliced

3 medium sized potatoes, chopped

2 turnips, chopped

1/4 cup fresh parsley, chopped very fine

2 tablespoons tomato paste

1 teaspoon black pepper

1 teaspoon kosher salt

1/4 cup lemon juice

1/4 teaspoon turmeric

1/4 teaspoon ginger

1/4 teaspoon saffron

1 1/2 cups dried chickpeas or garbanzos, soaked overnight

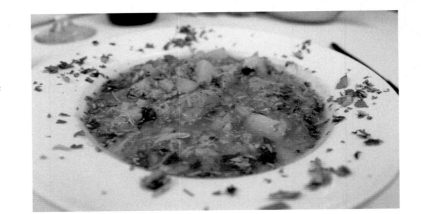

1. Place meat and veggies (except tomatoes) in a large saucepan. Add about 10 cups of water and bring to a boil.
2. Stir in tomatoes and tomato paste. Be very gentle and do not stir vigorously. You want the flavor to escape the tomatoes slowly.
3. Add chickpeas, spice and lemon juice. Slowly stir.
4. Reduce heat to low and allow to simmer for about 30-35 minutes covered or until meat and chickpeas are done.

BREADS

Pita Bread

Pita is a traditional Middle-Eastern flat bread. It is often served with spreads such as hummus, zaalouk, and bakoula, and is often used to make custom gourmet sandwiches.

¼ oz. (1 packet) dried yeast

1 ¼ cup of warm water

1 teaspoon of sugar

3 ½ cups of all-purpose flour

½ teaspoon of kosher salt

1 tablespoon of extra virgin olive oil

1. Dissolve the yeast in ¼ C of warm water. Add the Sugar and set in a warm place for 10-15 minutes until it becomes bubbly.
2. Sift the flour and salt together in a large mixing bowl.
3. Make a well in the center and pour in the yeast mixture. Knead by hand, gradually adding the remaining water, until a firm dough forms.
4. Continue kneading the dough for 10-15 minutes until it no longer sticks to your hands.
5. Knead in the olive oil.
6. Cover the bowl with a damp cloth and set in a warm place for 2 hours, or until doubled in size.
7. Punch the dough down, and knead for an additional 5 minutes.
8. Portion the dough into golf ball sized pieces. Flatten the dough balls with a rolling pin, or by hand, on a lightly floured board until they are about ¼ inch thick and around 6 inches in diameter.
9. Lay the rounds on a floured cloth. Cover them with another floured cloth and let them rise in a

warm place for another 20-30 minutes.

10. Preheat the oven to 500 degrees Fahrenheit.

11. Oil two baking sheets and place them in the oven for at least 10 minutes to preheat.

12. Sprinkle the dough rounds lightly with cold water and slide them onto the preheated baking sheets.

13. Bake for 6-10 minutes, or until the smell of fresh baked bread fills your kitchen. Do not let the Pita brown, it should be white and puffed.

14. Place the Pita on wire racks to cool.

15. Preferably, serve right away with a spread or as a sandwich. Pita can also be reheated as needed in a 450F oven for 2-3 minutes. Store leftovers in a plastic bag or wrapped tightly in foil.

Baguette

Morocco is a country rich in French influence. The classic baguette is a staple of many Moroccan meals. This soft yet crusty bread is baked fresh and served often with tajines, soups, and spreads.

¾ tablespoons (1 ½ packets) dry yeast

1 ½ cup of warm water

1 ½ teaspoon kosher salt

3 cups of all-purpose flour

1. Dissolve the yeast in ½ cup of the warm water, let sit for 15-20 minutes.
2. Dissolve the kosher salt in the rest of the warm water.
3. Sift the all-purpose flour into a large mixing bowl. Make a well in the center. Pour in the yeast mixture and mix lightly with the flour.
4. Add the Salt Water. Mix by hand until a dough forms. Turn the dough out onto a floured board and knead for 10-15 minutes, or until it no longer sticks to your hands.
5. Cover the dough with a cloth and let it rise in a warm place for one hour.
6. Preheat the oven to 400F. Knead the dough again for about 5 minutes. Divide it in half, and form each piece into a roll about 14 inches long (or the length of a sheet pan).
7. Place the two dough logs onto a floured sheet pan and let sit for 20 minutes.
8. Using a very sharp knife, make 4 diagonal slits on each loaf. Brush the loaves with cold water.
9. Place a small bowl of ice in the bottom of the oven.
10. Place the pan of dough on the middle oven rack. Bake the baguettes for 45 minutes to 1 hour, brushing with cold water every 15 minutes.
11. When the bread is lightly browned, remove from oven and set on wire racks to cool.

SIDE DISHES

Saffron Rice

6 cups of water

2 oz. vegetable base

Pinch of saffron threads

1 packet of saffron powder

3 c rice

1 tablespoon of extra virgin olive oil

1 teaspoon of kosher salt

2 tablespoons of butter, unsalted

1. Bring water, vegetable base, saffron threads, and saffron powder to a boil.

2. In a separate pot, combine rice, olive oil, and salt and cook over medium heat for 2 minutes.

3. Pour boiling stock over rice. Cover and cook for 25 minutes, or until liquid is absorbed and rice is tender.

4. Pour Rice onto a sheet pan, spread evenly and rub with butter.

Saffron Couscous

Saffron Couscous is a staple side dish in Moroccan cuisine, and is also used in quite a few other recipes, such as soups and salads.

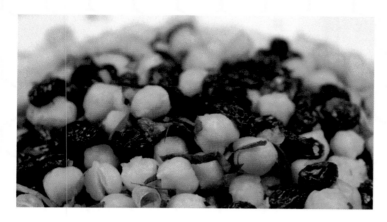

32 oz. Carton Vegetable Stock

1 Pinch Saffron Threads

2 C Couscous

½ T Olive Oil

1 tsp Kosher Salt

1. In a saucepan, bring the Vegetable Stock and Saffron threads to a boil.
2. In a large bowl combine the Couscous, Olive Oil, and Kosher Salt. Mix the Couscous and oil together with your hands, this will help to evenly distribute the oil and keep the grains from sticking together.
3. Pour the boiling stock over the couscous, give it one quick stir and let sit. No further cooking is required. The boiling stock is hot enough to cook the tiny grains of couscous just by letting it sit. Fluff well with a fork before serving.

Vegetarian Couscous Royal with Baked Vegetables in a Saffron & Herb Sauce

Ingredients:

1 onion cut in diced

1 zucchini sliced longwise

1 large carrot sliced longwise

1 sweet potato cubed

1 turnip cubed

1 red bell pepper cut in slices

1 cup chopped cabbage

1 cup chickpeas

3 tbsps. finely chopped fresh parsley

3 tbsps. finely chopped cilantro

2 tsps. paprika

2 tsps. turmeric

2 tsps. ginger

1 tsp sea salt

1 pinch saffron

3 tsp Olive Oil

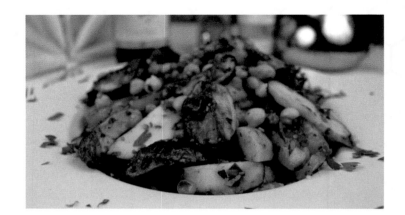

Steamed Vegetable Preparation:

Steamers come in a variety of forms. The stainless steel fold-up variety fits inside a pot to keep the vegetables above sauce. Some pots are specifically made with holes in the bottom for steaming over another pot of sauce. To steam vegetables, simply follow these steps:

1. Wash vegetables
2. Bring water to a boil
3. Add parsley, cilantro, paprika, turmeric, ginger, cayenne, salt, saffron, Olive Oil.
4. Place vegetables in a steaming basket over the sauce and cover

5. Steam until they become bright in color or have reached desired texture
6. Remove vegetables from pot and arrange them artistically on couscous or quinoa.
7. Serve the remaining sauce on the side, when is needed for more moisture to Quinoa (gluten free) or couscous. Or add red hot pepper to the sauce if you desire heat? For the meat Lovers add Chicken, lamb, beef, or fish, You can bake chicken or lamb in the vegetable sauce, and steam fish in the same sauce, serve the meat on the top of your Quinoa or couscous, and vegetable.

Couscous Preparation:

Prep Time: 2 minutes

Steam time: 5 minutes

Ingredients

1 Cup of couscous.
2 cups of boiled vegetable sauce from steamed vegetable.

Directions:

1. Combine couscous and vegetable sauce in a saucepan and Cover for 5 minutes

Quinoa Preparation: For people with Gluten intolerance.

Before cooking, quinoa must be rinsed to remove the toxic (but naturally occurring) bitter coating, called saponin. Saponin, when removed from quinoa, produces a soapy solution in water. Quinoa is rinsed before it is packaged and sold, but it is best to rinse it again at home before use. Place quinoa in a grain strainer and rinse thoroughly with water.

Prep Time: 2 minutes

Cooking Time: 15-20 minutes

Serves 4

Ingredients:

> 1 cup quinoa
> 2 cups vegetable sauce from steamed vegetable.

Directions:

1. Using a fine mesh strainer, rinse quinoa with cool water until the water runs clear.
2. Combine quinoa and vegetable sauce in a saucepan. Cover and bring to a boil.
3. Reduce heat to a simmer and continue to cook covered for 15 minutes or until all sauce has been absorbed.

Enjoy the whole food goodness!

Saffron "Grains"

In addition to the saffron rice and couscous, I will introduce you to a variety of exciting grains you may or may not be familiar with. Possibly some you've heard of or been curious about, yet were apprehensive to try. Cooking and eating should be pleasurable, as opposed to just seen as necessity. Have an adventure, venture out and try something new!

Grains are a great way to add some variety to some everyday meals. Here are basic instructions for preparing a variety of them in basically the same manner as you would the Saffron Rice or Saffron Couscous.

> 1 32 oz. Carton Vegetable Stock
>
> 1 Pinch Saffron Threads
>
> 1-2 C Grain of Your Choice (see chart for ratios of stock to grain)
>
> ½ T Olive Oil
>
> 1 tsp Kosher Salt

Follow the instructions on the chart for ratios and cooking times. Once you get comfortable preparing the grains using the simple saffron broth, do not be afraid to experiment. You could try adding different fresh or dried herbs. How about adding finely diced vegetables to make a pilaf?

Here are a few ideas to get started:

> *Quinoa with tiny diced Carrots, Potatoes, and Turnips*
> *Polenta with chopped Tomatoes and Fresh Basil*
> *Bulgar with crumbled Feta and Kalamata Olives*
> *Let your imagination and taste buds explore!*

Whole grains have been a central element of the human diet since early civilization. They are an excellent source of nutrition, as they contain essential enzymes, iron, dietary fiber, Vitamin E, and B-complex vitamins. Because the body absorbs grains slowly, they provide sustained and high-quality energy.

The quickest way to prepare great grains is to experiment and find what works for you. Remember one cup of dry grains yields 2 to 4 servings. Here are basic directions:

Measure the grain, check for bugs or unwanted material, and rinse in cold water using a fine mesh strainer.

Optional: soak grains for one to eight hours to soften, increase digestibility, and eliminate phytic acid. Drain grains and discard the soaking water.

Add grains to recommended amount of water and bring to a boil.

A pinch of sea salt may be added to grains to help the cooking process, with the exception of kamut, amaranth, and spelt (salt interferes with their cooking time).

Reduce heat, cover, and simmer for the suggested amount of time, without stirring during the cooking process.

Chew well and enjoy every bite!

1 Cup Grains	Water	Cooking Time	Contains Gluten?
Common Grains:			
Brown rice	2 cups	45-60 minutes	no
Buckwheat (aka kasha)*	2 cups	20-30 minutes	no
Oats (whole oats)	3 cups	75-90 minutes	questionable due to content, contact, or contamination
Oatmeal (rolled oats)	2 cups	20-30 minutes	questionable due to content, contact, or contamination
Alternative Grains:			
Amaranth	3 cups	30 minutes	no
Barley (pearled)	2-3 cups	60 minutes	yes
Barley (hulled)	2-3 cups	90 minutes	yes
Bulgur (cracked wheat)	2 cups	20 minutes	yes
Cornmeal (aka polenta)	3 cups	20 minutes	no
Couscous**	1 cup	5 minutes	yes
Kamut	3 cups	90 minutes	yes
Millet	2 cups	30 minutes	no
Quinoa	2 cups	15-20 minutes	no
Rye berries	3 cups	2 hours	yes
Spelt	3 cups	2 hours	yes
Wheat berries	3 cups	60 minutes	yes
Wild rice	4 cups	60 minutes	no

All liquid measures and times are approximate. Cooking length depends on how strong the heat is. It's a good idea, especially for beginners, to lift the lid and check the water level halfway through cooking and toward the end, making sure there is still enough water to not scorch the grains, but don't stir. Taste the grains to see if they are fully cooked. The texture of grains can be changed by boiling the water before adding the grains. This will keep the grains separated and prevent a mushy consistency. Cooked grains keep very well.

Brown Rice

Unlike white rice, brown rice has all bran layers intact and thus contains all of its naturally present nutrients. These layers of bran act to protect the grain and to help maintain its fatty acids. Brown rice contains the highest amount of B vitamins out of all grains. Additionally, it contains iron, vitamin E, amino acids, and linoleic acid. Brown rice is high in fiber, extremely low in sodium, and is composed of 80% complex carbohydrates.

Characteristics:

- Promotes good digestion
- Quenches thirst
- Balances blood sugar and controls mood swings

Buying & Storing:

Look for quality brown rice that contains a small amount of green grains. We recommend buying high quality organic brown rice and storing it in airtight glass jars in a dark cupboard.

Basic Brown Rice

Prep Time: 5 minutes

Cook Time: 45–60 minutes

Serves 4, yields 3 cups

Ingredients:

> 1 cup brown rice
> 2 cups of water or broth
> Salt or other seasonings to taste

1. Rinse rice in a bowl of cool water and strain.
2. Place all ingredients in a pot with a tight-fitting lid.
3. Bring to a boil, then reduce heat.
4. Cover and let simmer for 50 minutes. If you are not experienced with cooking rice, you'll want to check the rice 10 minutes before the anticipated finish time so you don't burn the rice. (If you do burn it, it is okay, just try it again!)
5. Remove from heat and let stand 10 minutes.
6. Fluff with fork and serve.

Saffron Millet

Millet is a very small, round grain with a history that traces back thousands of years. It was the chief grain in China before rice became popular and continues to sustain people in Africa, China, Russia, and India, among other places. Millet is an extremely nutritious and hardy crop that grows well under harsh or dry conditions, both of which contribute to its widespread use and popularity around the world.

Characteristics:

- Gluten-free
- High in protein, fiber, iron, magnesium, and potassium
- Contains silica, which helps keep bones flexible in aging process
- Soothing, especially for indigestion or morning sickness
- Anti-fungal; helps ease Candida symptoms
- Improves breath
- Warming; good to eat in cool or rainy weather
- Supports kidneys and stomach

Uses:

Millet can be used in porridges, cereal, soups, and dense breads. It is a delicious wheat-free substitution for couscous, as it has a similar consistency. In parts of Africa, millet is fermented to make beer.

Buying & Storing:

Look for yellow colored, raw millet in health food stores. Millet is often found in the bulk section of the health food store and is generally not sold in regular supermarkets. Store in an airtight jar or glass container for six to nine months.

Preparation:

Rinse millet before cooking, and use one-part millet to two parts liquid.

Basic Millet

Prep Time: 2 minutes

Cooking Time: 30 minutes

Serves 4

Ingredients:

> 1 cup millet
> 2 cups of water
> A few grains of sea salt

1. Rinse millet in a grain strainer.
2. Place all ingredients in a pot with a tight-fitting lid.
3. Bring to a boil, reduce heat to low.
4. Simmer 30 minutes.

Saffron Quinoa

Quinoa (pronounced KEEN-wah) has the highest nutritional profile and cooks the fastest of all grains. It is an extremely high energy grain and has been grown and consumed for about 8,000 years on the high plains of the Andes Mountains in South America. The Incas were able to run such long distances at such a high altitude because of this powerful grain.

Characteristics:

- Contains all eight amino acids to make it a complete protein
- Has a protein content equal to milk
- High in B vitamins, iron, zinc, potassium, calcium, and vitamin E
- Gluten-free; easy to digest
- Ideal food for endurance
- Strengthens the kidneys, heart, and lungs

Uses:

When quinoa is cooked, the outer germ surrounding the seed breaks open to form a crunchy coil, while the inner grain becomes soft and translucent. This double texture makes it delicious, versatile, and fun to eat. To save time, cook a lot of quinoa at once, and eat it as leftovers. Quinoa can be reheated with a splash of soy or nut milk for breakfast porridge; you can add dried fruit, nuts, and cinnamon for a sweet treat. Add finely chopped raw vegetables and dressing for a cooling salad, or add chopped, cooked, root vegetables for a warming side dish. Store dry, uncooked quinoa in a cool, dry, dark place in a tightly closed glass jar for up to one year.

Preparation:

Before cooking, quinoa must be rinsed to remove the toxic (but naturally occurring) bitter coating, called saponin. Saponin, when removed from quinoa, produces a soapy solution in water. Quinoa is rinsed before it is packaged and sold, but it is best to rinse again at home before use. Place quinoa in a grain strainer and rinse thoroughly with water.

Basic Quinoa

Prep Time: 2 minutes

Cooking Time: 15–20 minutes

Serves 4

Ingredients:

> 1 cup quinoa
>
> 2 cups water

1. Using a fine mesh strainer, rinse quinoa with cool water until the water runs clear.
2. Combine quinoa and water in a saucepan. Cover and bring to a boil.
3. Reduce heat to a simmer and continue to cook covered for 15 minutes or until all water has been absorbed.
4. Remove from heat and let stand for 5 minutes covered; fluff with a fork.
5. Season as you like.

***For a delicious toasted flavor, dry roast for 5 minutes in saucepan before adding liquid.**

Saffron Kasha

Kasha is the name for buckwheat that has been roasted to a deep amber color. It is one of the oldest traditional foods of Russia. Despite its name, buckwheat is not actually a member of the wheat family, but rather a relative of rhubarb. Of all the grains, buckwheat has the longest transit time in the digestive tract and is the most filling.

Characteristics:

- Stabilizes blood sugar
- Gluten-free
- Builds blood; neutralizes toxic acidic waste
- Benefits circulation
- Strengthens the kidneys
- High proportion of all eight amino acids, especially lysine
- Rich in vitamin E and B-complex vitamins

Uses:

Kasha has a strong, robust, earthy flavor and makes a very hearty meal. It can be eaten as a hot breakfast cereal, a side dish, or a grain entrée mixed with vegetables.

Preparation

The only way to cook kasha is to add it to boiling water. This keeps the grains separate and less mushy. It also makes the cooking process faster. Do not add kasha to cold water, as it will not cook properly.

Basic Kasha

Prep Time: 5 minutes

Cooking Time: 20 minutes

Serves 4

Ingredients:

> 1 cup kasha
> 2 cups water
> Pinch of sea salt

1. Bring water to a boil.
2. Slowly add kasha and pinch of sea salt.
3. Cover and let simmer 20 minutes.
4. Fluff with fork.

Kasha Sweet Potatoes

Prep Time: 5 minutes

Cooking Time: 20–25 minutes

Serves 4

Ingredients:

2 cups water

1 cup kasha

1 medium sized sweet potato, chopped small

1/4 cup of corn (fresh or frozen) chopped

1 small onion, diced

Pinch of sea salt

1 small zucchini, chopped

Tahini (optional)

1. Bring water to a boil.
2. Add chopped sweet potato and boil for 6 minutes.
3. Add onion, zucchini, corn, pinch of sea salt, and kasha.
4. Cover pot and reduce to a simmer.
5. Simmer for 15 to 20 minutes, and do not stir.
6. Fluff before serving. Enjoy!

Variation: Serve topped with a little bit of tahini.

Buckwheat (Kasha) Tabouli

2 C Vegetable Stock

1 Pinch Saffron Threads

1 C Buckwheat Groats (Kasha)

1 Medium-sized Cucumber, Diced

1 Large Tomato, Diced

½ C Green Onions, Finely Chopped

½ C Cilantro, Chopped

2 C Parsley, Chopped

1 tsp Garlic Puree

1 Fresh Lemon, Juice of

2 tsp Kosher Salt

½ C Olive Oil

1. In a saucepan, bring the Vegetable Stock and Saffron threads to a boil.

2. Add the Buckwheat (Kasha). Cover and reduce heat to medium-low. Simmer for 20 minutes.

3. Fluff with a fork and allow to cool to room temperature.

4. Mix the cooled Buckwheat (Kasha) with all of the other ingredients in a large bowl. Chill in the refrigerator for at least one hour (this will allow the flavors to mingle).

5. Serve as a salad on top of mixed green or as a side dish. Also, it can be topped with Chickpeas and crumbled Feta for a hearty vegetarian meal option.

Roasted Red Potatoes

2 lbs. small red potatoes

¼ cup extra virgin olive oil

2 tablespoons of oregano

Pinch of salt

1. Pre-heat oven to 425 degrees.
2. Wash potatoes and quarter, or dice into bite-size pieces.
3. Spread a thin covering of olive oil onto a large baking pan and arrange one layer of potatoes, cut side facing up, onto the pan.
4. Drizzle remaining olive oil over the potatoes, add a pinch of salt, and evenly sprinkle the oregano over all of the potatoes.
5. Roast in the oven for approximately 25 minutes: add time if needed until the potatoes are slightly browned and fork tender.

SAUCES

Moroccan Honey Sauce

4 oz. vegetable base

3 cups of water

1 pinch of pure Spanish saffron

1 packet of regular saffron

6 bay leaves

35 Cloves

5 cinnamon sticks

½ cup pure honey

1 tablespoon of garlic

1. In a large pot, bring all but the honey to a boil.
2. Add the honey and return to a boil.
3. When sauce rises to the top of the pot, heat at a low simmer for 10-15 minutes.
4. Add to mixture of lamb, vegetables, and fruits or other dish and simmer for another 10-15 minutes.

Charmoula

Zesty Cilantro and Parsley Pesto

1 large bunch of cilantro (coriander)

1 large bunch of parsley

8 cloves garlic

2 tablespoons of paprika

2 tablespoons of cumin

1 teaspoon of salt, or more to taste

¼ teaspoon saffron threads, crumbled

¼ cup of vegetable oil

3 tablespoons of red wine vinegar

Juice of 1 small lemon

1. Add garlic, spices, salt, oil, vinegar, and lemon juice to your food processor and blend until smooth.
2. Roughly chop the cilantro and parsley, add to the food processor, and blend for approximately 3 minutes (or longer, depending on your model of food processor) until the greens are finely shredded.
3. Enjoy as a marinade, on a sandwich, adding to your salads, or for flavoring bites of other dishes.
4. This sauce is magically used in Moroccan cuisine, you can use it as the Main base ingredient in all your seafood Tajines.

Cinnamon-Citrus Carrot Dip

10 cups Carrots

10 cups of water

1 cup Charmoula (see page 82)

1 lemon, juiced

1tbsp cinnamon

1/2 cup brown sugar

Preparation...

In a large pot bring water to a boil. Add carrots and boil and cook until soft.

Drain water.

Combine all remaining ingredients in food processor, add boiled carrots and purée.

Place carrot dip in a large bowl and refrigerate for 30 minutes.

Serve with raw vegetables; broccoli, celery and cauliflower.

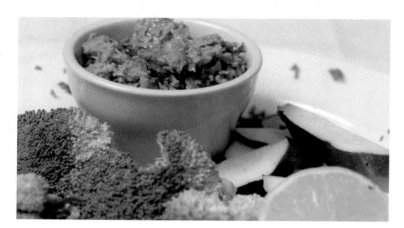

Lemon Basil Vinaigrette

½ cup of lemon juice

½ cup of red Wine Vinegar

1 cup Olive Oil

1 tablespoon Salt

½ cup fresh basil

Combine all ingredients in a blender and mix until emulsified.

Tatziki

Yogurt–Cucumber Sauce

1 tub of plain (preferably Greek-style) yogurt

¼ cup of water

2 tablespoons of lemon juice

1 tablespoon of oregano

Pinch of kosher salt, to taste

1. Empty contents of the tub of yogurt into a large mixing bowl.
2. Add water, lemon juice, oregano, and a pinch of salt.
3. Mix well. Add more salt and / or oregano to taste.
4. Enjoy on a sandwich or as a dipping sauce for meats or salads.

ENTREES: SEAFOOD

Mahi Mahi with Black Olives

Two 8 ounce portions of fresh Mahi Mahi

I cup of diced fresh tomato

3 tbsps. Charmoula (see page 82)

4 tbsps. of diced Moroccan black olives

2tsp olive oil

1/2 cup of water

Salt, to taste

Preparation:

Preheat oven to 350 degrees.

In a large baking pan combine 1/2 cup water and 2 tsp. olive oil, then place Mahi Mahi.

Bake for 25 minutes.

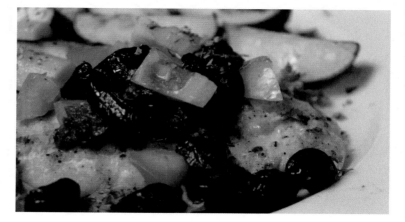

Bruschetta prep:

In a sauce pan over medium heat cook tomatoes with Charmoula and olives, about 10 minutes.

Pour Bruschetta over Mahi Mahi.

Serve it with a roasted potato and Enjoy!

Moroccan Crabcakes

Makes 8 servings:

1 lb. fresh (or canned) lump Maryland crab

8 tbsps. Charmoula (see page 82)

1 egg

3/4 cup semolina flour

4 tbsps. of organic grass fed butter or ghee

2 lemons, cut into 8 slices for garnishing each crab cake

Preparation:

Makes eight 2 ounce crab cakes.

In a large mixing bowl combine all ingredients (except butter/ghee and lemon) stirring together with a spatula and mix well.

In a large pan over medium heat add 2 tbsps. of butter or ghee and let melt before adding crab cakes.

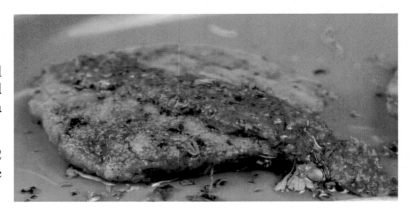

Use hands to create four 2 ounce crab cake patties then place each into pan and sear, approximately 5 minutes on each side, or until golden brown.

Repeat for the remaining four crab cakes.

Plate crab cakes and top with Charmoula sauce and slice of lemon.

Pilpil

Stewed shrimp & scallops in a zesty cilantro pesto, served with warm bread

Makes 2 servings.

>   1 cup or 6 tiger shrimp
>   2 cups bay scallops
>   1/2 cup Charmoula (see page 82)

Preparation...

Place all ingredients in a medium sized sauce pan and simmer over medium heat, stirring occasionally until shrimp are pink with firmly curled tails. Bay scallops should be cooked when this happens. Be careful not to over-cook shrimp and scallops.

Serve in a small tajine or bowl with crispy bread for dipping.

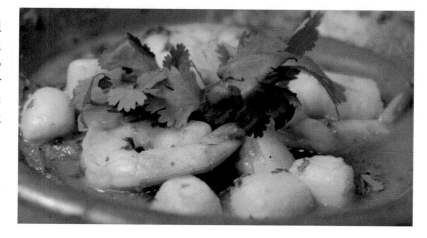

>   2 tbsps. olive oil
>   1-2 tbsps. water

Saffron Mussels

2 lbs. fresh Prince Edward Island Mussels

2 cups heavy cream

1 tsp puréed garlic

2 tsp dry basil

I pinch Saffron

Preparation...

Over medium heat, combine all ingredients. Cover the pan.

As the mussels steam check to see that all mussel shells have opened, stir and reduce the cream sauce around the opened mussels.

Place mussels and all sauce in a large bowl.

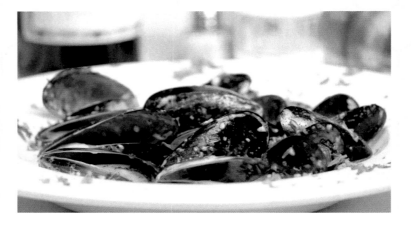

Seafood Paella

6 cups of water (for Saffron rice prep)

10 cups of water (for Seafood prep)

2 oz. vegetable base

Pinch of saffron threads

3 cups of rice

1 tablespoon of extra virgin olive oil

1 teaspoon of kosher salt

2 tablespoons of organic grass fed butter or ghee

1 cup fresh carrots, thickly sliced

1 cup peas

1 cup Charmoula (see page 82)

1 lb. fresh mussels

1 lb. tiger shrimp, peeled and de-veined

1/2 lb. bay or sea scallops

8 ounces Halibut, cut in 3 inch pieces

8 ounces Mahi Mahi

Preheat oven to 350 degrees.

In a separate large baking pan combine all ingredients -10 cups of water, 1 cup of Charmoula, olive oil, salt, butter or ghee, along with peas, carrots, fish, shrimp and scallops.

Cover pan with baking pan lid and cook for 30 minutes or until all seafood is cooked and all mussels have opened.

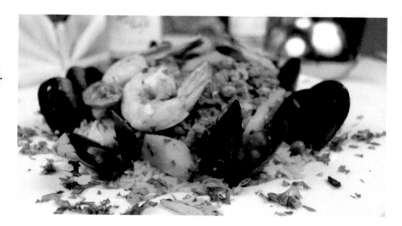

Stuffed Grouper With Spinach And Ricotta Cheese Served With Couscous And Mixed Sautéed Vegetables

Two servings: 4 Grouper fillets, approximately 4 ounces each

> 1 cup Bakoula (see page 48)
>
> 1 cup ricotta cheese
>
> 1 cup Charmoula (see page 82)
>
> 3/4 cup water
>
> 3tbsp olive oil
>
> 1 tbsp. paprika
>
> Sprinkle of sea salt, to taste
>
> KOSHER salt

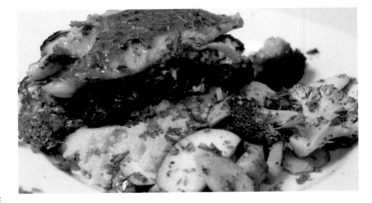

Preparation:

Preheat oven to 350 degrees.

On a baking sheet place 2 fillets of grouper side by side with about 2 to 3 inches in between.

Spread your first layer, a 1/2 cup of Bakoula, onto each of the grouper fillets.

On top of the layer of Bakoula spread a 1/2cup of ricotta cheese for the second and final layer.

The remaining two grouper fillets are then placed on top of the ricotta cheese to complete each 'stuffed' grouper.

Add water to the baking sheet all around the stuffed fillets, then drizzle olive oil over the top of the fish.

Sprinkle with paprika and sea salt.

Serve stuffed baked grouper with Charmoula on top.

Recommend to be served atop Saffron couscous and steamed vegetables tossed with oregano.

ENTREES: POULTRY

Moroccan Honeyed Cornish Hen

2 Cornish hens

¼ cup lemon juice

1 large onion, sliced

2 cloves garlic, finely diced

2 pinches saffron

1 teaspoon black pepper

Kosher salt, to taste

1 tablespoon ginger

4 dried prunes

4 dried apricots

1 pear, peeled and halved

1 cup honey

2 teaspoons cloves

1 tablespoon cinnamon

2 tablespoons sesame seeds

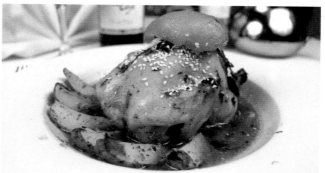

1. Preheat oven to 450 degrees.

2. Rinse Cornish hens with fresh water and lemon juice, then sprinkle with salt. Rub hens with garlic, ginger, black pepper and 1 pinch saffron. Drizzle with extra-virgin olive oil.

3. Pour 1 cup water in baking pan; add onions. Cover with lid and bake for 1 hour.

4. Place a saucepan half full of water on stove. Add the other pinch of saffron with cloves, salt, honey, garlic and cinnamon. Bring to a boil, stirring.

5. When mixture has come to a boil, add apricots, prunes and pears. Simmer for 15 minutes.

6. Remove from stove and add mixture to pan with Cornish hens. Bake 5 to 10 minutes more.

7. To serve, place each hen in a tajine. Cover with one pear and honey onion; add sauce as needed. Place two apricots and two prunes on each side of Cornish hens. Sprinkle with sesame seeds.

* A Tajine is a decorative, ceramic Moroccan pot with a lid used to serve meat stews. If you do not own a tajine, you can use any vessel with a lid safe to use on a stovetop.

Ginger Chicken Tajine

4 chicken halves

Lemon juice

1 large onion, thinly sliced

2 cloves garlic, finely diced

2 pinches saffron

1 teaspoon black pepper

Kosher salt, to taste

2 tablespoons ginger

2 tablespoons parsley, roughly chopped

½ cup peas

2 carrots, sliced diagonally

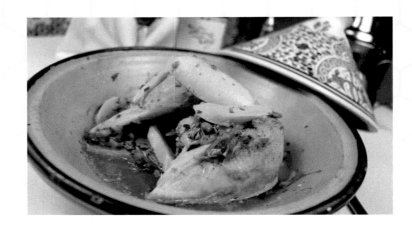

1. Preheat oven to 450 degrees.
2. Rinse chicken halves with fresh water and lemon juice; sprinkle with salt. Rub chicken with garlic, ginger, black pepper, parsley and 2 pinches saffron.
3. Pour 1 cup water in baking pan; add onions. Cover with lid and bake for 1 hour.
4. Place a saucepan half full of water on stove. Add ginger, saffron, salt, and garlic. Bring to a boil, stirring.
5. When mixture has come to a boil, add carrots and peas. Simmer for 15 minutes.
6. Remove from stove and add mixture to pan with chicken. Bake 5 to 10 minutes more.
7. To serve, place each chicken half in a tajine or large bowl. Add saffron broth with peas and carrots. Place preserved lemon on top of chicken as garnish. Sprinkle with parsley.

Chicken Bastilla

Chicken halves

1 handful bleached almonds

¼ cup butter

8 eggs

Phyllo dough, 8 large sheets

1 tablespoon of ground cinnamon

¼ cup honey

Powdered sugar, sprinkle to taste

Saffron broth from Ginger Chicken Recipe (see page 92)

Sugar, to taste

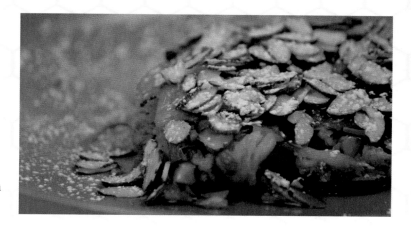

1. Take Chicken halves from Saffron sauce. In a large cooking pan, collect the Ginger Chicken Saffron sauce.

2. Whisk together 8 eggs, adding sugar and cinnamon, to taste. Stir until dry.

3. Take two baked chicken halves and peel the meat from bone, chop with kitchen knife.

4. Deep fry bleached almonds and grind in blender to medium texture.

5. To close bastilla in an 8" cooking pan, lay down phyllo dough on pan, brushing each layer with melted butter. Pad with scrambled egg mixture. Next cover with chopped chicken and finish with ground almonds.

6. Close with phyllo dough and cut to portion. Roast in 350-degree oven for 10 minutes. Remove from oven and serve on dessert plate, drizzle with honey and sprinkle with powdered sugar and cinnamon.

Cumin Chicken Tajine

4 chicken halves

Lemon juice

1 large onion, thinly sliced

Whole bulb garlic, finely diced

2 pinches saffron

1 teaspoon black pepper

Kosher salt, to taste

2 tablespoons of ginger

4 tablespoons of cumin

2 tablespoons parsley, roughly chopped

2 fresh tomatoes, diced

4-6 medium sized potatoes, peeled and cut into wedges

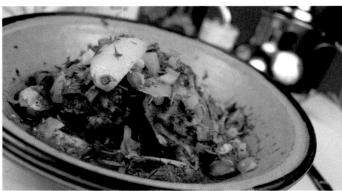

1. Preheat oven to 450 degrees.
2. Rinse chicken halves with fresh water and lemon juice; sprinkle with salt. Rub chicken with half of your garlic, 1 tbsp. ginger, and 2 tbsps. cumin, black pepper, parsley and 2 pinches saffron.
3. Pour 1 cup water in baking pan; add onions. Cover with lid and bake for 1 hour.
4. Place a saucepan half full of water on stove. Add remaining 1 tbsp. ginger, remaining 2 tbsps. cumin, 1 pinch of saffron, pinch of salt, and remaining garlic. Bring to a boil, stirring.
5. When mixture has come to a boil, add potatoes and tomatoes. Simmer for 15 minutes.
6. Remove from stove and add mixture to pan with chicken. Bake 5 to 10 minutes more.
7. To serve, place each chicken half in a tajine or large bowl. Add saffron-cumin broth with tomatoes and potatoes. Place preserved lemon on top of chicken as garnish. Sprinkle with parsley.

Saffron Chicken Tajine With Cauliflower

4 chicken halves

Lemon juice

Whole cauliflower, cut into florets

1 large onion, thinly sliced

2 cloves garlic, finely diced

2 pinches saffron

1 tsp of cardamom

1 teaspoon black pepper

Kosher salt, to taste

2 tablespoons ginger

2 tablespoons parsley, roughly chopped

1. Preheat oven to 450 degrees.

2. Rinse chicken halves with fresh water and lemon juice; sprinkle with salt. Rub chicken with garlic, ginger, black pepper, parsley and 2 pinches saffron.

3. Pour 1 cup water in baking pan; add onions. Cover with lid and bake for 1 hour.

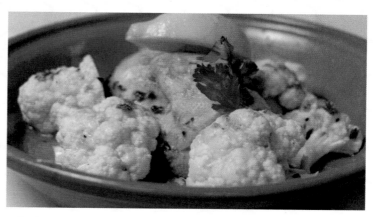

4. Place a saucepan half full of water on stove. Add cardamom, ginger, saffron, salt, and garlic. Bring to a boil, stirring.

5. When mixture has come to a boil, add cauliflower. Simmer for 15 minutes.

6. Remove from stove and add mixture to pan with chicken. Broil chicken, uncovered, 5 to 10 minutes more.

7. To serve, place each chicken half in a tajine or large bowl. Add saffron-cardamom broth with cauliflower. Place preserved lemon on top of chicken as garnish. Sprinkle with parsley.

ENTREES: LAMB

Lamb Tajine

4 pounds leg of lamb, cut into 4 oz. pieces

4 bulbs garlic, peeled and pureed in extra-virgin olive oil

4 onions, peeled and thinly sliced

1 teaspoon black pepper

Kosher salt, to taste

2 tablespoons ginger

Fresh parsley, chopped, to taste

Fresh cilantro, chopped, to taste

Cold pressed olive oil

1/3 cup sunflower oil

2 tablespoons coriander

½ cup peas

Artichoke hearts, for garnish

1. Prepare the lamb by trimming all fat and sinew. Cut into 4-oz. pieces.
2. Place lamb chunks in a pan and cover with garlic, salt, ginger, coriander, parsley, cilantro, black pepper and olive oil.
3. Toss everything together and let marinate, preferably overnight.
4. In a large pot, bring water to a boil. Add garlic, saffron, onions, parsley, cilantro, and ginger.
5. Bring pot to a boil.
6. Remove lamb from marinade and toss in flour to coat.
7. In a large sauté pan, heat vegetable oil. Fry lamb for 7-10 minutes or until browned on all sides.
8. Place browned lamb into pot of sauce. Simmer for 1 -1½ hour or until tender.
9. When lamb is done, add peas and artichoke hearts. Simmer for 10-15 more minutes until peas and artichokes are cooked.
10. Serve garnished with pickled lemon and accompanied by warm bread.

Honeyed Lamb with Pears

4-pound leg of lamb, cut into 4 oz. pieces

4 bulbs garlic, peeled and pureed in extra-virgin olive oil, divided

1 teaspoon black pepper

Kosher salt to taste

2 tablespoons ginger, divided

Fresh parsley, chopped, to taste, divided

Fresh cilantro, chopped, to taste, divided

¼ cup extra-virgin olive oil

1/3 cup vegetable oil

2 tablespoons coriander, divided

Pinch of saffron

4 onions, peeled and thinly sliced.

1 cup of dried pitted prunes

2 pears, peeled and cut into wedges

4 apricots, pitted, peeled and cut into wedges

2 cups of Moroccan Honey Sauce (see page 81)

1. Trim all fat and sinew from the lamb. Cut into 4 oz. pieces.

2. Place lamb chunks in a pan and cover with garlic, salt, saffron, ginger, coriander, parsley, cilantro, black pepper and olive oil.

3. Toss everything together and let marinate, preferably overnight.

4. In a large pot, bring water to a boil. Add garlic, saffron, onions, parsley, cilantro, and ginger.

5. Bring to a boil.

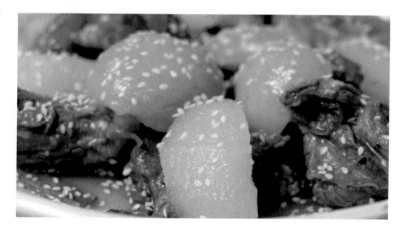

6. Remove lamb from marinade and toss in flour to coat.

7. In a large sauté pan, heat vegetable oil. Fry lamb for 7-10 minutes or until browned on all sides.

8. Place browned lamb into pot of sauce. Simmer for 1 -1½ hour or until tender.

9. When lamb is done, remove from cooking sauce. Place in Honey Sauce* along with pear halves, apricots, and prunes.

10. Serve garnished with pickled lemon and accompanied by warm bread.

Traditional Boneless Lamb with Peas and Artichokes

4 pounds leg of lamb, rinsed and cut into 4 oz. pieces

4 onions, peeled and thinly sliced

4 bulbs garlic, peeled and pureed in extra-virgin olive oil, to taste

2 tablespoons ginger

2 tablespoons coriander

12 oz. peas

16 pieces of artichoke hearts

Fresh parsley, chopped, to taste

Fresh cilantro, chopped, to taste

1 pinch saffron

Kosher salt, to taste

Fresh ground black pepper, to taste

In a large sauté pan, add the lamb. Pour in enough water or broth to cover the meat and brown the lamb on all sides. Discard all but 2 tablespoons of fat from the pan and reserve the broth.

To a separate pan over medium heat, add 2 onions and the garlic. Stir often, until the onions become limp, 3-5 minutes.

To the pan, add the ginger and coriander. Stir until fragrant, about 30 seconds.

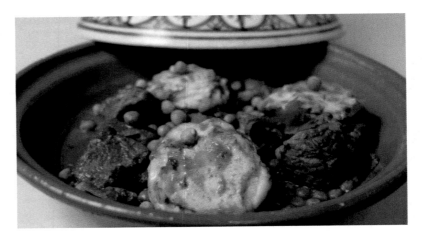

Turn the heat to high and add the chopped parsley and cilantro, to taste, as well as the saffron and half of the lamb to the broth. Bring to a boil. Reduce heat, cover and simmer, stirring occasionally, until the lamb is tender when pierced, about 1 hour. Skim off and discard any fat. Add salt and pepper, to taste.

Add artichoke hearts and peas and cook with lamb for another 15 minutes.

Serve the lamb mixture in a ceramic tajine topped with 2 artichoke hearts and peas. Garnish with a wedge of pickled lemon and serve with warm fresh bread.

Chef Sentissi's Traditional Lamb M'Rosia

There's a saying around Saffron Café, "Mmmmmm... M'Rosiaaaa!" And for a wonderfully delicious reason: A 16 ounce bone-in New Zealand lamb shank slow-roasted for 2 hours in a rich & hearty vegetable purée sauce of onions, potatoes, carrots & garlic prepared with the sweet and spicy flavors of honey, nutmeg, & cinnamon along with the deeper flavors of ginger & clove - all balanced with lots of saffron & just a touch of cayenne… Sweet & spicy perfection!

2 lamb shank	2 pinches saffron	1 teaspoon cloves
1 Lb. onion, sliced	1 tablespoon oregano	1 tablespoon cinnamon
1 Lb. carrots	1 teaspoon black pepper	
2 Lb. potatoes		1 tablespoon cayenne
2 cloves garlic, diced	1 pinch Kosher salt	1 bunch shopped parsley
	1 tablespoon ginger	

1. Preheat oven to 450 degrees.
2. In Blender puree 1Lb carrots and1Lb potatoes.
3. Place lamb shanks in baking pan, salt and rub with garlic, ginger, black pepper and 1 pinch saffron.
4. Add vegetable puree, cayenne, and cinnamon.
5. Drizzle with extra-virgin olive oil, than add sugar.

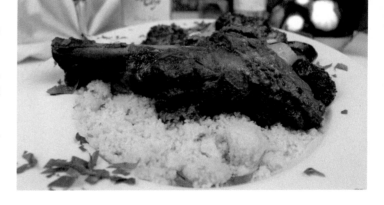

6. Pour 1 cup water in baking pan; add onions. Cover with lid and bake for 1:30 hour at degrees.
7. Cut 1Lb of potatoes - quartered; place them on flat sheet pan, drizzle with extra- virgin olive oil and sprinkle with oregano. Bake for 25 minutes at 550 degrees.
8. To serve: place each shank in a tajine. Cover with vegetable puree; add sauce as needed. Place roasted potatoes on each side of shank. Garnish with pickled Lemon.

** A Tagine is a decorative, ceramic Moroccan pot with a lid used to serve meat stews. If you do not own a Tagine, you can use any vessel with a lid that is safe to use on the stovetop

ENTREES: BEEF

That's a Spicy **Mediterranean** *Meatball!*

1 lb. of ground beef or lamb

4 cloves of garlic, minced

1 teaspoon of kosher salt

½ white onion, finely chopped

¼ cup cilantro, finely chopped

1/8 cup parsley, finely chopped

½ teaspoon of cinnamon

1 teaspoon of paprika or cayenne pepper

½ teaspoon of ground ginger

½ teaspoon of fresh ground black pepper

2 egg yolks

Knead ground beef until soft.

Add the egg yolks and mix together until soft. Add all listed spices and seasonings, the onion, cilantro, and parsley. Knead until evenly mixed.

Roll ground beef and spice mixture into meatballs, 2 inches long by one-inch wide.

Grill until thoroughly cooked. Enjoy!

Kafta – Another Preparation

There are many forms of Kafta found throughout the Middle-East and Mediterranean region. It is similar to sausages or burgers in other parts of the world. Kafta is traditionally made from either ground beef or lamb, and full of an exciting array of spices. Kafta is typically grilled and served either on a sandwich or stewed in a tajine with vegetables and eggs then served with fresh hearty bread.

1 lb. Ground Beef

¾ T Paprika

¾ T Ginger

2 tsp Coriander

2 tsp Cumin

1 Pinch of Nutmeg

1 Pinch of Black Pepper

¾ tsp Cinnamon

2 T Garlic Puree

¼ tsp Kosher Salt

1 ½ tsp Olive Oil

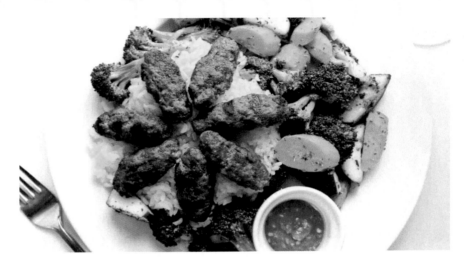

1. Combine all of the ingredients in a large bowl.

2. Wet your hands and begin to knead the meat and spices together. Continue mixing until all of the spices are fully absorbed by the meat and a paste has formed.

3. Roll the Kafta (using wet hands) into small sausage like pieces about 2 inches long. The Kafta can also be shaped into small patties if you prefer.

4. Grill the Kafta over medium heat turning every 2 minutes until no pink is visible. (Kafta, as well as all ground meats, should reach an internal temperature of 165F).

5. Serve on warm bread with lettuce, tomato, Pickled Onions, Harissa, and Yogurt Sauce. Kafta is also delicious served on top of Saffron Rice or Couscous.

Andalusian Style Spicy Beef Stew

2 ¼ lb. Lean Beef (rump steak or other firm cut), cut into Cubes

1 Green Bell Pepper, cut into Strips

1 Large Tomato, cut into Wedges

1 Onion, Sliced

2 Carrots, Peeled and Diced

3 Potatoes, Peeled and Sliced

1 Head of Garlic

1 Bay Leaf, Fresh if you can find it

1T Parsley, Minced

1 Whole Clove

1 Small Piece Stick Cinnamon

1 Pinch Saffron Threads

½ T Kosher Salt

6 Black Peppercorns

8 Olive Oil

1. Roast the head of Garlic under the broiler or on a grill for about 10 minutes, turning frequently. Let cool. Separate and peel the cloves.

2. Heat 4 T of the Olive oil in a large pot with a lid. Brown the Beef in the Olive Oil.

3. Add the Bell Pepper, Tomato, Onion, and Carrots. I tried this recipe with different verities of vegetables, always you discover different flavors and deliciousness.

4. In a mortar or spice grinder, crush the Peppercorns with the Clove and Cinnamon. Add the Roasted Garlic and mash into a paste. Blend in the Saffron.

5. Add 1C Hot Water to the paste and mix. Pour this mixture into the pot with the Beef and Vegetables.

6. Add the additional 4 T Olive Oil, Bay Leaf, and Parsley. Sprinkle with ½ T Kosher Salt. Cover the pan and simmer for 45 minutes.

7. Add a little bit more hot water if it is too thick for your liking.

Add the peeled and sliced Potatoes. Taste and a bit more Kosher Salt if necessary. Replace the cover on the pan and simmer for another 25-30 minutes. Serve hot.

ENTREES: VEGETARIAN

Andalusian Style Artichokes and Eggs

4 Large Artichokes

4 Whole Eggs + 1 Egg Yolk

2 Lemons

½ tsp Cumin

1 T Mint, Chopped

4 Small Thyme Sprigs

4 T White Wine Vinegar

1 C Olive Oil

2 T Kosher Salt.

1. Trim the Artichokes, removing the stems and tough outer leaves. To keep them from darkening, place them in a bowl of cold water with the juice of 1 Lemon.

2. Sprinkle the Kosher Salt into a large pot of water and bring to a boil. Add 2 T White Wine Vinegar to help tenderize the Artichokes. Boil the Artichokes for 20-25 minutes, or until easily pierced with a fork. Drain and dry the Artichokes upside down, gently pressing down to help separate the leaves.

3. Beat the Egg Yolk with the juice from the other Lemon, Cumin, and Olive Oil until it forms a dense sauce. Set aside.

4. Poach the remaining 4 Eggs. Using the boiling water from the Artichokes, carefully break the Eggs, one at a time, into the water. Use a spoon to help keep the whites cloaked around their yolks. Lower the heat and simmer for about 3 minutes, until the eggs hold together but are still soft in the center.

5. Spread the leaves in the center of each Artichoke so that little "nests" form. With a slotted spoon, carefully remove the Eggs from the water and place one in each "nest".

6. Drizzle a spoonful of the sauce on top of each Egg. Garnish with Fresh Mint and a sprig of Thyme. Serve the remaining sauce in a dish so that your guests can help themselves to more if needed.

DESSERTS

Baklava

2 cups almonds

2 cups pistachios

2 tablespoons sesame seeds

1 cup sugar

Phyllo dough, 1 package (9-10 large sheets)

1 lb. butter, melted

½ cup honey

1 pinch of salt

1 teaspoon cinnamon

¼ cup sesame seeds

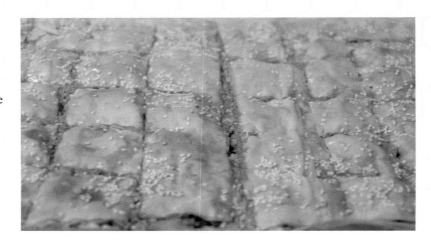

1. Chop almonds and pistachios using a food processor. Mix with 2 tablespoons of sesame seeds.

2. Toast nuts and seeds in the oven for about 5 minutes.

3. In a bowl, combine nuts, sesame seeds, sugar, butter, honey, salt, and cinnamon. Mix well.

4. Rub a thin layer of melted butter on a half size sheet pan (14"x18"). Place two sheets of phyllo on top buttered pan.

5. Place 1/3 of the nut mixture onto phyllo. Place two more layers of phyllo on top of nuts. Spread with butter. Repeat 2 more times with other 2/3 of nut mixture.

6. Place two layers of phyllo on top, spread with melted butter and sprinkle with sesame seeds. Repeat until all phyllo is gone, ending with a phyllo layer. Brush with melted butter.

7. Cut into 3-inch squares.

8. Bake at 375 for 10-12 minutes.

Enjoy!

Tiramisu

3 (3 oz.) packages of lady finger cookies

½ cup strongly brewed coffee, room temperature

6 egg yolks

1 cup of sugar

1 (16 oz.) tub of mascarpone cheese

1 quart of heavy cream

2 tablespoons of unsweetened cocoa powder

2 tablespoons of rum or Italian Marsala (optional)

Pinch of salt

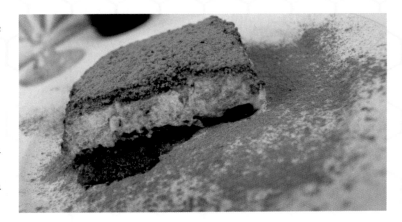

1. Prepare the coffee, add 2 tablespoons of sugar (or sweeten to taste) and cool to room temperature.
2. Combine the egg yolks, sugar, mascarpone cheese, cream, salt, and rum (optional) in your food processor. Blend until creamy and fluffy.
3. Dip the lady finger cookies in the coffee mixture so they are lightly soaked yet maintain their firmness.
4. Layer half of the cookies on a baking pan, then layer one half of the cream mixture on top.
5. Repeat with another layer of cookies, then the rest of the cream on top.
6. Sprinkle with cocoa powder.
7. Cover the pan with plastic wrap and refrigerate for at least 3 hours so the flavors can soak in and the tiramisu can settle.

Enjoy!

Fragrant Moroccan Orange Salad

4 fresh oranges

1 tablespoon of cinnamon

1 tablespoon of powdered sugar

2 tablespoons of orange blossom water

1. Peel oranges and dice into bite-size pieces.
2. Add the cinnamon, powdered sugar, and orange blossom water. Toss lightly until well mixed.

BEVERAGES

Honey-Mint Lemonade

Capture the essence of the summer sun and the natural goodness it brings in this healthy beverage. I like to combine fresh honey with fresh-squeezed lemon juice to this old-time favorite summer refresher.

Ingredients:

1 cup fresh squeezed lemon juice	2 cups purified water
1/2 cup honey	4 cups ice cubes
7 sprigs fresh mint	

(Makes 6 servings)

Instructions:

1. Place the lemon juice, honey, and 1 chopped sprig of the mint in a large pitcher and stir, pressing the mint and to release mint flavor.
2. Add the water and stir until the honey dissolves, then add the ice.
3. Pour into six 10-ounce glasses and garnish each glass with a sprig of mint and a fancy straw.

Tip:

Children three years old and younger can become seriously ill from honey, so please don't give them a glass of this lemonade. However, you can use local honey to help battle against seasonal allergies for older children and adults. Honey's thick coating, with the vitamin C in lemons combine perfectly to soothe a sore throat, relieve an upset stomach, or to help treat a cold.

Green Detox Juice:

1 bunch organic kale

1 organic cucumber

1 cup organic parsley

2 celery stalks

1 organic lemon

1 green apple

1 thin slice of ginger root

Green Energy Smoothie

1 cup water/coconut water

2 bunches organic kale

Juice of 1 lemon

1 organic green apple

1 frozen banana

2 organic pitted dates

1 – 2 slices of ginger root and Ice

Add a Protein—soaked almonds, protein mix or Chia Seeds

Acknowledgements

Sourcing was done out of the following literature and websites:

http://saffroncafeindy.com/

http://en.wikipedia.org/wiki/Garlic

http://en.wikipedia.org/wiki/Saffron

http://www.greenmedinfo.com/blog/ancient-saffron-magical-healing-powers-confirmed-science

http://www.gsk.com/research/how-we-discover-new-medicines.html

http://en.wikipedia.org/wiki/History_of_medicine

http://www.ancient.eu.com/medicine/

http://www.merriam-webster.com/dictionary/medicine

http://www.ncbi.nlm.nih.gov/pmc/articles/PMC3684452/

http://www.forbes.com/sites/matthewherper/2013/08/11/the-cost-of-inventing-a-new-drug-98-companies-ranked/

http://www.forbes.com/sites/matthewherper/2013/08/11/how-the-staggering-cost-ofhttp://www.takingcharge.csh.umn.edu/explore-healing-practices/food-medicine/how-does-food-impact-health-inventing-new-drugs-is-shaping-the-future-of-medicine/

http://www.foodbycountry.com/Kazakhstan-to-South-Africa/Morocco.html

http://www.takingcharge.csh.umn.edu/explore-healing-practices/food-medicine/how-does-food-impact-health

http://en.wikipedia.org/wiki/Moroccan_cuisine

http://www.wafin.com/articles/39/The-secret-of-the-Moroccan-diet

http://www.fao.org/ag/agn/nutrition/mar_en.stm

http://www.eatingwell.com/food_news_origins/food_travel/a_taste_of_morocco

http://www.journeybeyondtravel.com/news/morocco-travel/morocco-food.html

We serve authentic Moroccan dishes and offer cooking classes in our upscale restaurant. Feeling like some Moroccan Mediterranean Food? Get your favorites at Saffron Cafè Make your reservation online:

http://saffroncafeindy.com/

Everything we do at Wholestic Nutrition is centered around you—because you hold the keys to shaping your own health. To know more about us, visit the link below.

https://wholesticnutrition.com/ For other book by Author, you can purchase from the link below:

Functional Nutrition Medicine Weightloss Program.: THE CUTTING EDGE SCIENCE FOR LOSING WEIGHT NUTRITION THAT ACTIVATES THE BODY, MIND & SPIRIT - Kindle edition by Dr Anass Sentissi, Functional Medicine University. Health, Fitness & Dieting Kindle eBooks @ Amazon.com.

https://www.amazon.com/Functional-Nutrition-Medicine-Weightloss-Program-ebook/dp/B07JB974XD

Printed in the United States
By Bookmasters